GOOD CHOLESTEROL, BAD CHOLESTEROL

HOW TO ORDER:

Quantity discounts are available from the publisher, Prima Publishing & Communications, P.O. Box 1260GBP, Rocklin, CA 95677; telephone (916) 786-0426 . On your letterhead include information concerning the intended use of the books and the number of books you wish to purchase.

U.S. Bookstores and Libraries: Please submit all orders to St. Martin's Press, 175 Fifth Avenue, New York, NY 10010; telephone (212) 674-5151.

GOOD CHOLESTEROL,
BAD CHOLESTEROL

Eli M. Roth, M.D., F.A.C.C.

Sandra L. Streicher, R.N.

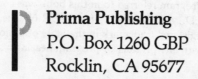

Prima Publishing
P.O. Box 1260 GBP
Rocklin, CA 95677

Editing by Helen Duncanson
Typography by R. Nolan & Sons
Production by Bookman Productions
Cover design by The Dunlavey Studio

Prima Publishing & Communications
Rocklin, CA

Library of Congress Cataloging-in-Publication Data
Roth, Eli.
  Good cholesterol, bad cholesterol.

  Bibliography: p.
  Includes index.
  1. Coronary Heart Disease—Prevention—Popular works.
  2. Atherosclerosis—Prevention—Popular works.
  3. Hypercholesteremia—Prevention—Popular works.
  4. Blood cholesterol.   5. Low-cholesterol diet.
  I. Streicher, Sandra. II. Title.
  RC685.C6R686 1988   616.1'2305   88-31625
  ISBN 1-55958-025-9

93 RRD 10 9 8 7 6 5 4

Printed in the United States of America

The HEARTSMART™Program referred to in this book was copyrighted in 1986 by Eli M. Roth, M.D., and Sandra L. Streicher, R.N. The name HEARTSMART™is a registered trademark in the State of Ohio and is not associated in any way with any product or program bearing a similar name.

Dedication

We dedicate this book to our parents and our children. The goal of learning from the past is to improve the future. As our parents taught us what they felt was proper, we hope to teach each of our children how to live healthy and heartsmart lives. The extensive time and effort that went into this book will not be in vain if at least one other person benefits from its contents.

Preface

There is now no question that cholesterol is linked to heart disease. Multiple studies have shown a direct relationship between abnormal cholesterol levels and increased risk of heart disease. More important, several studies in recent years have shown that decreasing cholesterol levels do result in a lower incidence of heart attack. It is for this reason that the public has been bombarded with cholesterol information. As a cardiologist and cardiovascular nurse, we are all too familiar with the result of elevated cholesterol—heart attack, stroke, and weakening and blockages in other arteries (atherosclerosis). Our patients have asked for easy to read, understandable information about cholesterol. They wanted something other than a list of "Do's and Don'ts" and needed information and advice that could be used for a lifetime—not a temporary "fad diet." We searched for this type of information, and were unable to find it in any one source. There is a great deal of cholesterol information available, but we feel this book is the first to bring it all together in a readable, easy to understand, medically correct form. This book gives accurate information and provides basic behavior modification principles which make lifetime eating habit changes possible. *Good Cholesterol, Bad Cholesterol* will not only explain what to do, but it will help you to understand why. A great deal of time and effort went into the research and writing of this book. We feel that the end result reflects our efforts and that the book does fulfill the goals which we set.

EMR and SLS

Foreword

Coronary artery disease today remains the number one cause of death in the United States.

The public seems infatuated with spectacular cases of the total artificial heart and transplantation in dealing with endstage coronary artery disease. However, seemingly as unpopular as it may appear, the much more effective means of combatting coronary artery disease is in the prevention of the disease by the adaptation of lifestyle.

Good Cholesterol, Bad Cholesterol provides a comprehensive source of information on cholesterol in an easily understood fashion. The book explains the physiological impact of cholesterol and the significance of its management and control. The authors furnish an account of different types of lipids in the blood and types of dietary fats. There is an informative chapter on label reading and an explanation of how the blood lipid levels are tested, as well as the current National Institutes of Health and American Heart Association recommendations.

This book provides a general overview of how to obtain and maintain recommended lipid levels and discusses the different medications used to treat lipid disorders not manageable with dietary alterations only. The reader is afforded with practical information on hints for dining out in restaurants and some recipe ideas.

I believe this book offers the general public a valuable insight into the benefits of a disease preventative lifestyle.

WILLIAM C. DEVRIES, M.D.

Contents

1   Why Worry About Cholesterol?

Why should anyone worry about something they really can't see, let alone understand? Was Mom wrong when she told you to eat your eggs and bacon so you would grow up to be big and strong? According to the American Heart Association, 1.5 million people will suffer a heart attack in the coming year and of those, more than 500,000 people will die. Heart attacks are caused by coronary artery disease (blockages in the blood vessels supplying blood to the heart). Elevated blood cholesterol is a major cause of these blockages. In addition, these blockages can and do form in any of the arteries in the body (also known as atherosclerosis). This can lead to stroke, high blood pressure, blood supply problems to the legs, or aneurysm (a weak spot or bulging in the arteries).

Fortunately, by controlling the blood cholesterol level, formation of these blockages can be slowed or even stopped. Over the past seventy-five years there have been many research studies that clearly prove elevated blood cholesterol levels cause an increase in atherosclerosis and coronary artery disease. Then why has the fuss over cholesterol just occurred in the last few years? Because, until recently, no study proved that lowering the blood cholesterol levels would reduce the risk of developing coronary artery disease and a heart attack. The Lipid Research Clinics Coronary Primary Prevention Trial (LRC CPPT) was a study that proved without a doubt, that lowering cholesterol levels did lower the risk of heart attack. This study was conducted by the National Institutes of Health and is considered the most important medical study on cholesterol to date. The study took ten years to complete, was conducted in twelve centers in North America, involved 3,806 men*, and cost $150 million. The results of the LRC CPPT proved beyond a doubt that lowering the blood cholesterol *does* lower the risk of suffering a fatal or nonfatal heart attack. The results of ten years of follow-up in these men demonstrated that for every 1% the blood cholesterol is lowered, the risk of heart attack is lowered 2%! In other words, two groups of men who were identical as far as age, weight, smoking, blood pressure, etc. were compared to each other. These groups, which started identical and stayed identical other than cholesterol level, had a marked difference in the occurrence of heart attack. For example, a man in the cholesterol controlled group who lowered his cholesterol blood level 10% had a 20% less chance of a heart attack than if he had not lowered his cholesterol.

So what are you waiting for? Reduce your blood cholesterol level and reduce your chance of heart disease. Since most of the cholesterol in the blood comes from food containing cholesterol, or more important, saturated fats,

---

*The National Institutes of Health Consensus Development Conference Statement on Lowering Blood Cholesterol to Prevent Heart Disease states: "This benefit of lowering cholesterol has been demonstrated most conclusively in men with elevated blood cholesterol levels, but much evidence justifies the conclusion that similar protection will be afforded to women with elevated levels."

learning how to control and modify your eating is the first step to lower cholesterol. This book will teach you to understand and conquer cholesterol. You will learn what your recommended cholesterol level should be, how to have the cholesterol level in the blood properly checked, and what medications your physician can prescribe to help lower the cholesterol level if proper diet alone is not sufficient. Most importantly, you will understand cholesterol enough when you finish this book to make dietary management easier as well as practical and palatable. You will learn how to eat as if your life depends on it.

CHOLESTEROL AND CARDIOVASCULAR DISEASE

Cholesterol is a major contributing cause of cardiovascular disease. Cardiovascular disease is a general term that is used to describe problems with the blood vessels or heart. Approximately 63 million Americans have some form of cardiovascular disease and atherosclerosis is the most common form. Atherosclerosis is a progressive condition that affects the arteries or "tubes" that carry blood, oxygen and nutrients to the body as well as to the heart itself. As the heart pumps, or beats, it moves the blood through these tubes. Normally, the inside of the arteries are smooth, and they expand and contract with each heartbeat as the blood flows through them. But in atherosclerosis there is a build-up of cholesterol, fat, and calcium within the smooth inside lining of the artery. This build-up gradually becomes hardened. For this reason atherosclerosis is frequently called hardening of the arteries. Not only does atherosclerosis cause the inside of the artery to narrow so that less blood can flow through, it also decreases the ability of the artery to expand and contract.

The arteries that supply the heart with blood are called the coronary arteries. When the coronary arteries are affected by atherosclerosis, the heart does not receive the blood supply it needs, and the result could be a heart attack. The development of atherosclerosis is dependent upon the build-up of cholesterol, fats, and other substances within the arteries. Therefore, if you reduce the amount of cholesterol and fats in the blood, you will decrease the development and progression of atherosclerosis. The best way to begin to reduce the blood cholesterol level is to limit the amount of cholesterol in your diet and modify the kinds of fats you eat.

2 Lipids, Cholesterol, and Triglycerides

There are so many different terms that people use when talking about cholesterol that it can become confusing. Before we start with how to control your cholesterol, let's get a better understanding of these terms and the language of cholesterol.

What are lipids? Lipids are fats. Lipid is the most general term used to describe all of the fats within the body. The body needs certain amounts and kinds of fats to function properly. Just as oil and water do not mix, lipids (oil) and blood (water) will not mix. For lipids to be transported in the bloodstream and put to use in the body, they combine with proteins. These lipid-protein combinations are called lipoproteins. Since fats combine with proteins to do the work that is required of them, the terms lipid and lipoprotein for all practical purposes mean the same thing. The general category of lipids is made up of several different kinds of fats. As you will see and understand, some lipids cause the development and progression of atherosclerosis, while other lipids are actually helpful in preventing atherosclerosis.

One category of blood lipids is cholesterol. Our understanding of cholesterol and specifically the different types of cholesterol has increased tremendously over the past several years. Cholesterol can be divided into two major types. The first type is the Low Density Lipoprotein cholesterol. It is known as LDL cholesterol. *LDL is the bad cholesterol.* LDL cholesterol is the fat that enters the inside lining of the artery and causes atherosclerosis. The second type of cholesterol is the High Density Lipoprotein cholesterol. This is known as HDL cholesterol. *HDL is the good cholesterol.* This particular kind of cholesterol actually fights against atherosclerosis and the build-up of fat in the arteries. There are other types of cholesterol but the two major groups are LDL and HDL.

Another group of blood lipids is known as triglycerides. Currently, triglycerides are less well understood than cholesterol. However, research has shown a correlation between elevated triglyceride levels and an increased incidence of atherosclerosis. In general, cholesterol appears to be a much more important factor in the development of atherosclerosis than triglycerides.

To review, the term lipid or lipoprotein refers to any fat in the body. The primary kinds of lipids in the blood are cholesterol and triglycerides. Within the category of cholesterol we have two major types, the bad cholesterol known as LDL and the good cholesterol known as HDL.

WHERE DOES CHOLESTEROL COME FROM?

Cholesterol is actually an important substance that is used in the production of many different body tissues and hormones. Because of its importance, your body has the ability to produce or synthesize cholesterol. Cholesterol which is produced by the body is said to be "endogenous."

All animals (as well as fish and fowl) produce and utilize cholesterol within their bodies. The majority of cholesterol in your body actually comes from eating (ingesting) foods which contain cholesterol and saturated fat. This will be explained further in Chapter 3. These foods are mainly of animal origin. Cholesterol which is obtained from outside sources is termed "exogenous." The total amount of cholesterol the body requires is relatively small. Therefore, most of the cholesterol found in the blood is more than the body needs. This excess cholesterol in the blood enters the walls of the arteries and forms deposits or plaques and the beginning of atherosclerosis. When these plaques are in the arteries providing the blood supply to the heart, the atherosclerosis causes coronary artery disease. Since a major portion of the cholesterol within the bloodstream is from exogenous sources, limiting cholesterol and saturated fat intake will normally have a significant effect on lowering blood cholesterol levels. The lowering of blood cholesterol levels has been shown to slow the progression of atherosclerosis and coronary artery disease.

NORMAL LEVELS VERSUS RECOMMENDED LEVELS

In the last several years, we have learned that there is a definite difference between the "normal" and "recommended" levels of cholesterol in the blood. The levels of cholesterol which have been considered "normal" for a long time are actually too high and are above the newer "recommended" blood cholesterol levels. Simply stated, the American public has had high cholesterol levels for quite some time. These high levels are almost always secondary to the usual American diet which is high in cholesterol and saturated fats. The blood cholesterol levels which were considered normal in the past are really an average (or mean) of blood cholesterol levels found in a wide cross-section of people. These levels were never correlated with the occurrence of atherosclerosis or coronary artery disease until recently. The newer "recommended" levels are based on the levels of risk of developing coronary artery disease. The "Desirable Blood Cholesterol" level is less than 200 mg./dL. Cholesterol levels of 200–239 mg./dL are considered "Borderline-High Blood Cholesterol" and greater than 240 mg./dL is considered "High Blood Cholesterol." If the blood cholesterol level is within the borderline-high range, then dietary changes should be initiated to lower the cholesterol level. If the level is above the high-risk level, then diet modification is attempted first. When diet alone is not successful, medication to lower cholesterol should be used. In general, the lower the blood cholesterol level, the less the chance of development of coronary artery disease. More detailed information about the recommended levels will be given in Chapter 6.

BLOOD CHOLESTEROL LEVELS	
Less than 200 mg./dL	Desirable
200 – 239 mg./dL	Borderline–High
Greater than or equal to 240 mg./dL	High

3 Understanding Fats in Food

Various types of fats are found in many of the foods you eat, and your body uses these fats in totally different ways. The three basic categories of dietary fats found in food are cholesterol, "saturated fats," and "unsaturated fats." Eating cholesterol rich foods will obviously increase your blood cholesterol level. Ingesting saturated fats also raises your blood cholesterol level whereas unsaturated fats will actually lower your cholesterol level. For this reason it is important for you to understand and recognize each category. Information on cholesterol in foods as well as cholesterol dietary recommendations will be covered in Chapter 4. The remainder of this chapter will deal with saturated and unsaturated fats.

Saturated fats raise the blood cholesterol level, and this in turn causes the development and progression of atherosclerosis. Therefore, you want to limit the intake of saturated fats in your diet. How can you tell if a product contains saturated fat? Examining the product label may tell what kind of fats are contained in the food. (This will be covered in Chapter 5.) Many foods are now labeled with not only the total fat content, but also the specific amount of saturated fat. If the label does not tell you the saturated fat content, There are two rules of thumb to follow to determine if saturated fats are present. The first rule is that saturated fats are solid at room temperature. The second rule is that dairy products and any food made from animal sources are high in saturated fats. (This may make more sense if you remember that milk is from an animal source.) Two exceptions to these rules are palm and coconut oils. Although these oils are from vegetable sources and can be in liquid form, both are high in saturated fat.

To help reduce the amount of saturated fat in your diet, you must avoid or limit foods that are high in saturated fats. This would include solid shortenings, fatty meats, products made from animal fats, and dairy products *with a high butterfat content.* Butter, cream, and whole milk contain cholesterol as well as saturated fats. Therefore, anything made from these dairy products contains both saturated fat and cholesterol. Some examples of this are ice cream, cheese, and baked goods. The saturated fat content of dairy products can be lowered. Whole milk contains 3.5% butterfat. The lower butterfat content is signified by a percent in the labeling, such as 2%, 1%, or .5%. To make a wise low-fat food choice you would pick the milk product with the lowest butterfat content. The American Heart Association recommends the use of .5% milk (skim milk is .5% or lower) for all adults of children over two years of age.

In summary, saturated fats are one type of fat found in the foods you eat. Saturated fats raise the cholesterol level in the blood and should be limited in your diet. Saturated fats are usually solid at room temperature and are found in foods from animal sources and dairy products. Palm and coconut oils are also high in saturated fat and should be avoided.

Let's see how the two rules of thumb about saturated fats can help you decide if a product is a wise low-fat choice.

Is lard a saturated fat? The answer is yes. It is a solid at room temperature, and it is made from animal products. Both of the rules of saturated fats apply to lard.

Does whole milk contain saturated fat? Yes, whole milk is a dairy product so according to the second rule it does contain saturated fat. Whole milk has a high butterfat (saturated fat) content.

Is liquid corn oil high in saturated fat? No. Corn oil is liquid at room temperature and is made from vegetable as opposed to animal sources. (It does not contain the exceptions of palm or coconut oil.)

Does "all vegetable shortening" contain saturated fat? The answer is yes. Although the shortening is made from vegetable sources, it is a solid at room temperature. The first rule tells you it is a saturated fat. Generally, the term "shortening" refers to a solid form whereas "oil" refers to a liquid form. *Many solid vegetable products are advertised as "Cholesterol Free" or "Contains No Cholesterol." These statements are true. They do not contain cholesterol, but they do contain saturated fat which raises the cholesterol level in your blood.* That is why it is so important for you to understand all of the factors that go into controlling your cholesterol.

Does "non-dairy coffee creamer" contain saturated fat? The answer will depend on the type of "non-dairy creamer" you use. Powdered non-dairy creamers almost always contain palm and/or coconut oil, and therefore, contain saturated fat. Liquid non-dairy creamers, such as Mocha Mix and Coffee Rich are made with soybean oil and therefore do *not* contain saturated fats.

WHAT ARE POLYUNSATURATED FATS?

Another type of fat found in the foods you eat is called polyunsaturated. The polyunsaturated fats tend to lower the cholesterol level in the blood. They do this by enabling the body to eliminate newly formed cholesterol that is excessive. Polyunsaturates are found in fish oils and liquid oils made from vegetables. *Once again, the exceptions to this are palm and coconut oils.*

Polyunsaturated fats can be changed to become solid at room temperature. This process is known as *hydrogenation.* When a polyunsaturated fat has been hydrogenated, it behaves like a saturated fat in the body and causes an increase in the blood cholesterol level. Foods may either be partially or completely hydrogenated. Many of the liquid vegetable oils are partially hydrogenated to produce margarine and other products. Foods containing oil that has been partially hydrogenated may be an acceptable low-fat food. In general, *completely hydrogenated oils should be considered as saturated fats.* The way to identify a good low-fat food choice is to read the label. If the food contains twice as much polyunsaturated as saturated fat, it is considered acceptable. Saturated fats raise the blood cholesterol level twice as much as an equal amount of polyunsaturated fat lowers the blood cholesterol level. By following the 2:1 ratio of polyunsaturated-:saturated, the blood cholesterol level will remain unchanged. By consuming more polyunsaturates than this, the blood cholesterol may actually be lowered.

EXAMPLES OF POLYUNSATURATED VEGETABLE FATS

Corn oil	Soybean oil
Sunflowerseed oil	Cottonseed oil
Safflower oil	Liquid all vegetable oil

Fish Oil Polyunsaturated Fats

Within the category of polyunsaturated fats are the vegetable fats, which we have just discussed, and fish oils. For many years little attention was paid to polyunsaturated fish oils. Then in the 1970's, a very important study examined the rarity of heart disease among the Eskimos in Greenland. This study found that their diet was limited almost exclusively to fish and fish products. It was interesting to the researchers that people who ate oily fish had virtually no heart disease. Because of this observation, fish oils were closely examined. Scientists have discovered that the polyunsaturates found in some cold-water, deep-sea fish are very effective in lowering blood cholesterol. It is now recognized that these polyunsaturated fish oils may lower cholesterol as do the vegetable polyunsaturates. But it is difficult to ingest enough fish oils in food to lower cholesterol level significantly. For this reason, companies are manufacturing fish oils in capsule or gelatin form that can be taken as a dietary supplement.

Vegetable and Fish Oil Polyunsaturates

About now you're probably asking yourself, "What's the difference between vegetable polyunsaturates and fish oil polyunsaturates since they both lower the blood cholesterol level?" That's a good question. The primary differences are in the chemical structure and in the way the body utilizes the fat, based on that chemical structure. Fats are made up of complex chains of fatty acids that occur naturally. In most *unsaturated* fats the first double bond (the unsaturated area) occurs in a certain position along the fatty acid chain. This position is called omega-6. Vegetable polyunsaturates are desaturated in this omega-6 position. However, fish oils are desaturated in a different area, the omega-3 position. This simple difference in desaturation position makes a difference in how fish oil and vegetable oil help lower blood cholesterol levels. In addition, the fish oils are longer in length and generally more unsaturated than the vegetable oils. Fish oils are especially rich in a long-chain omega-3 fatty acid known as EPA (eicosapentaenoic acid). We mention all of these names because the manufacturers of fish oil supplements are using these terms to make up names for their products. Some examples of these names are ProMega, ProtoChol, Cardi-Omega 3, and MaxEPA.

Table 3.1 Sources of Omega-3 Fatty Acids in Foods
(per 100 grams raw edible portion)

Food	Omega-3 Fatty Acids (gm)	Cholesterol (gm)
Cod liver oil	19.2	570
Salmon oil	20.9	485
Bass (fresh water)	0.3	59
Cod (Atlantic)	0.3	43
Halibut (Pacific)	0.5	32
Mackerel (Atlantic)	2.6	80
Perch (white)	0.4	80
Salmon (pink)	1.0	-*
Tuna (albacore)	1.5	54
Trout (lake)	2.0	48
Crab (Alaska king)	0.3	-
Shrimp (Atlantic)	0.3	142
Clam (soft shell)	0.4	-
Walnut oil	10.4	0
Butternuts (dried)	8.7	0
Soybean oil	6.8	0
Walnuts (black)	3.3	0
Beans (common, dry)	0.6	0
Strawberries	0.1	0

*A dash indicates the lack of data available for nutrient known to be present.
Adapted from F.N. Hepburn et al: Journal American Dietetic Association 86:794, 1986

Again, the body's use of any substance is dependent upon its chemical structure. In this case, the omega-3 position appears to be a more potent agent for reducing blood cholesterol than the omega-6 position. The longer length of the omega-3 fatty acid chain and the increased number of desaturated areas within the chain (double bonds) may also be important factors in the fish oils' ability to lower cholesterol. Interestingly, the fish and fish oils that are high in omega-3 polyunsaturates are also high in cholesterol. As you have just learned, ingesting cholesterol will raise your blood cholesterol level. Despite this high cholesterol content, the omega-3 polyunsaturates still cause an overall lowering of the blood cholesterol level. This suggests that they are a potent 'cholesterol-lowering agent. In addition, several of the fish oil supplements are now cholesterol-free due to special processing. If fish oil supplements are used, these cholesterol-free supplements are recommended. There is still controversy as to the benefit of fish oil and fish oil supplements in lowering cholesterol. We recommend that you consult with your physician or dietician if you are considering the use of fish oil supplements. Remember that polyunsaturated fats from any source lower blood cholesterol.

In Table 3.1 we have listed some foods that are high in omega-3 fatty acids. Notice the high cholesterol content of the fish sources.

ALL POLYUNSATURATED FATS AND OILS ARE NOT CREATED EQUAL

All of the oils and fats that you eat contain saturated, polyunsaturated, and monounsaturated fats. Monounsaturated fats are a special type of polyunsaturate. They contain only one (mono) double bond, instead of many (poly) double bonds found in the polyunsaturated fats. Previously it was believed that monounsaturated fats did not lower or raise the blood cholesterol level. Recently, several studies have suggested that monounsaturates do indeed lower the blood cholesterol level. In fact, monounsaturates may lower the LDL (bad) cholesterol level without affecting the HDL (good) cholesterol level. These same blood cholesterol. For this reason you will want to choose oils that have the highest percent of polyunsaturated fat. All fats and oils contain 9 calories/gram (see Chapter 4), so caloric intake will not be a factor in the type of oil you choose. Listed below are some oils and fats with the percent of saturated and polyunsaturated fats they contain. Because monounsaturated fats do not lower the blood cholesterol, a polyunsaturated fat is preferred. Peanut, canola and olive oils are true monounsaturates. We have given the monounsaturated fat content of a few of the oils for you as examples, but the saturated/polyunsaturated fat ratio is the important factor.

Type of Oil/Fat	Percent Polyunsaturated Fat	Percent Saturated Fat
Safflower Oil	74%	9%
Sunflower Oil	64%	10%
Corn Oil	58%	13%
Vegetable Oil (soybean and cottonseed)	40%	13%
Peanut Oil	30%	19%
Chicken Fat (Schmaltz)	26%	29%
Olive Oil	9%	14%
Vegetable Shortening	20%	32%
Lard	12%	40%
Beef Fat	4%	48%
Butter	4%	61%
Palm Oil	2%	81%
Coconut Oil	2%	86%

Type of Oil	Percent Polyunsaturated	Percent Monounsaturated	Percent Saturated
Olive Oil	9%	77%	14%
Peanut Oil	30%	51%	19%
Safflower Oil	74%	17%	9%
Sunflower Oil	64%	26%	10%
Corn Oil	58%	29%	13%
Canola Oil	32%	62%	6%

4 Your Daily Intake of Cholesterol and Fats

An apple a day may not keep the doctor away, but the American Heart Association thinks the right amount of cholesterol and the proper kinds of fat will help keep heart disease away. Now that you understand the different kinds of fats and can recognize the good types from the bad ones, it's time to put all of this into daily practice. The recommendations from the National Institutes of Health and the American Heart Association apply to all Americans over the age of two. Their recommendations are as follows:

1. The total intake of dietary fats should be reduced to 30% of total daily calories.

2. The 30% of calories from fats should be divided as follows: less than 10% saturated fat (less than $1/3$ of total fat); no more than 10% polyunsaturated fat (up to $1/3$ of total fat); 10–15% monounsaturated fat ($1/3$ to $1/2$ of total fat).

3. Reduce total daily intake of cholesterol to 250–300 mg. or less.

4. Total daily calorie allowance should be reduced to correct obesity and maintain ideal body weight.

The dietary restrictions as listed above constitute what is referred to as the **Step 1 diet**. The Step 1 diet is recommended for all Americans over the age of two and is consistent with good nutrition. The Step 1 diet is the first step on the way to controlling cholesterol. If further restrictions in the diet are necessary to reduce blood cholesterol to the recommended levels, there is a **Step 2 diet**. The Step 2 diet is to be followed only on the advice of a physician and with the counseling of a dietician. The Step 2 diet restricts the total fat intake to less than 30%, as does Step 1. The Step 2 diet, however, limits saturated fat intake to less than 7% of total calories. (Step 1 diet is less than 10% for saturated fat intake.) Step 2 diet restricts the intake of cholesterol to less than 200 mg. per day; whereas, the Step 1 diet recommends less than 300 mg. of cholesterol per day in the diet.

Since the Step 1 diet is the recommendation for the general public, we will be examining how to incorporate the Step 1 diet into your daily eating habits. If you must progress to the Step 2 diet on the recommendation of your physician, you will continue to apply the very same guidelines that will be described in this book, but with stricter limitations.

In order to apply these recommendations, there are some facts you need to know and some calculations you will need to make. First, you must know (or calculate) your average daily intake of calories. The daily intake of calories by Americans is widely variable. The recommendation for adult females is between 1200 and 1800 calories per day. For adult males, the recommended intake is between 1600 and 2200 calories per day. Secondly, you need to know that one gram of fat provides 9 calories. For your information, one gram of protein provides 4 calories as does one gram of carbohydrate. You can see that gram for gram, fat contains twice as many calories as does carbohydrate or protein. This ability to provide more calories for less weight makes fat the body's most efficient method of long-term energy storage.

Once you know your average daily calorie intake, you can calculate your 30% allowable calorie intake from fats by multiplying by .30%. For example, if your daily calorie intake was 1800 calories, your allowable calorie intake from fat would be 30% of 1800 (.30 × 1800) or 540 calories. To find the number of grams of fat this is equal to, you would divide by 9, since each gram of fat equals 9 calories. In this same example, 540 calories of allowable fat intake would equal 540 ÷ 9) 60 grams of fat. The recommended intake of saturated fats is less than one-third of the calories due to fat. In this example, you could take 1/3 of the total fat allowance of 60 grams to obtain 20 grams, so the allowable saturated fat is less than 20 grams. In the same way, the suggested polyunsaturate allowance is up to 1/3 of the total fat allowance or up to 20 grams. The remaining 1/3 to 1/2 of allowable fat is recommended to be monounsaturated. In this example, the monounsaturated fat would again be 20 to 30 grams. On food labels found in stores, fat content will be given in grams (not calories) when the fat content is listed. You can calculate the number of calories in a product due to fat by multiplying fat content in grams by 9 (calories). Some labels will specify the amount of saturated and polyunsaturated fats, although this is not currently required. Without this breakdown of saturated and polyunsaturated fat, it is difficult to know if you are meeting the specific 1/3 saturated, 1/3 polyunsaturated recommendation. To show how these recommendations work, we have some examples on the following pages. There is also a worksheet for you to figure the daily calories, cholesterol, and percent of fats in your diet.

The following are examples to show you how to calculate daily allowance of cholesterol and fats. You will have to use the worksheet on the following page to arrive at the amounts and percentages for yourself.

EXAMPLE 1

A man who eats an average of 2000 calories per day

Total Daily Calorie Intake: 2000

Total Daily Cholesterol Allowance: 250–300 mg.

Total Daily Fat Allowance = 30% of total calories or .30 × 2000 = 600 calories or 600 ÷ 9 = 66.6 grams of fat

Maximum Saturated Fat: less than 1/3 of the total allowable grams of fat or 1/3 of 66.6 = less than 22.2 grams of saturated fat

Polyunsaturated Fat: up to 1/3 of total allowable grams of fat or up to 22.2 grams

Monounsaturated Fat: 1/3 to 1/2 of the total allowable grams of fat = 22.2-33.3 grams

EXAMPLE 2

A woman who averages 1500 calories per day

Total Calorie Intake: 1500

Total Daily Cholesterol Allowance: 250–300 mg.

Total Daily Fat Allowance: 30% of total calories = .30 × 1500 = 450 calories or 450 calories ÷ 9 = 50 grams

Maximum Saturated Fat: less than 1/3 of total fat allowance = 1/3 × 50 grams = less than 16.6 grams

Polyunsaturated Fat: up to 1/3 of total fat allowance = 1/3 × 50 grams = up to 16.6 grams

Monounsaturated Fat: 1/3 to 1/2 of total fat allowance = 16.6 to 25 grams

EXAMPLE 3

An individual who eats 1800 calories per day

Total Calorie Intake: 1800

Total Daily Cholesterol Allowance: 250–300 mg.

Total Daily Fat Allowance: 30% or 540 calories
or 60 grams

Maximum Saturated Fat: less than $1/3$ of 60 grams =
less than 20 grams

Polyunsaturated Fat: up to $1/3$ of 60 grams =
up to 20 grams

Monounsaturated Fat = $1/3$ to $1/2$ of 60 grams =
20-30 grams

DAILY CHOLESTEROL AND FAT ALLOWANCE WORKSHEET

(Unsaturated Fats include Polyunsaturated and
Monounsaturated)

Breakfast

Food	Calories	Total Fat	Sat.	Unsat.	Chol.

Totals: _____ _____ ___ _____ _____

Lunch

Food	Calories	Total Fat	Sat.	Unsat.	Chol.

Totals: _____ _____ ___ _____ _____

Dinner

Food	Calories	Total Fat	Sat.	Unsat.	Chol.

Totals: _____ _____ ___ _____ _____

Snacks Throughout the Day

Food	Calories	Total Fat	Sat.	Unsat.	Chol.

Totals: _____ _____ ___ _____ _____

	Calories	Total Fat	Sat.	Unsat.	Chol.
Breakfast Total:	_____	_____	___	_____	_____
Lunch Total:	_____	_____	___	_____	_____
Dinner Total:	_____	_____	___	_____	_____
Snack Total:	_____	_____	___	_____	_____
Daily Total:	_____	_____	___	_____	_____

STEP 1
Daily Total Fat Allowance in Calories =
Total Calories × .30

STEP 2
Daily Total Fat Allowance in grams = (Step 1) ÷ 9

STEP 3
Maximum Daily Saturated Fat Allowance in grams =
less than (Step 2) × $^1/_3$

STEP 4
Maximum Polyunsaturated Fat Allowance in grams
= up to (Step 2) × $^1/_3$
Maximum Daily Cholesterol Allowance =
250-300 mg.

STEP 5
Monounsaturated Fat Allowance = (Step 2) × ($^1/_3$ to $^1/_2$)

5 Reading and Understanding Labels

This chapter will concentrate on providing guidelines to help in the process of selecting low cholesterol and low saturated fat food choices. In the first four chapters you have learned what cholesterol is, where it comes from, and how the body utilizes it. You have also learned about the different types of cholesterol and how each type either accelerates or retards atherosclerosis and heart disease. The recommended daily allowances for dietary intake of fats and cholesterol as well as the normal and recommended blood levels have been discussed. Since *dietary control is the key* to the entire issue of conquering cholesterol, it is extremely important that you be able to practice what you have learned and will learn. Now it is time to put all of your cholesterol knowledge to work for you. In this chapter, you will learn how to make wise cholesterol selections based on food groups in combination with reading and interpreting labels.

In selecting any food, you want to consider its cholesterol and saturated and unsaturated fat content. Saturated fats actually have more effect on the blood cholesterol level than does dietary cholesterol. The best dietary control of your cholesterol requires limiting foods high in cholesterol and saturated fats, while increasing the foods high in unsaturated fats. We will start with some broad guidelines for categories of food. Vegetable sources of food, with the exception of palm and coconut products, are always lower cholesterol choices than animal products. If you are choosing animal products, fish is the best choice. Turkey and chicken without the skin are the next best. (Remember to remove the skin from the turkey and chicken, because that is where the largest amount of cholesterol and saturated fat is contained.) When choosing beef, pork, or veal, remove as much fat as possible *before* cooking. If you cook with the fat on the meat, the fat will be absorbed into the meat. Trimming fat after cooking is not an efficient way to be in control of cholesterol. Dairy products are also a source of cholesterol and saturated fat. Low-fat dairy foods include skim milk and .5% milk, nonfat yogurt, ice milk (if it does not contain palm or coconut products), mozzarella cheese, and buttermilk made from skim milk. These low-fat products would be good choices as well as substitutions for the dairy products you currently use. Dairy products moderately high in cholesterol and saturated fats include 1% or 2% milk, low-fat cottage cheese, and yogurt.

Dairy products that are high in cholesterol and saturated fat include whole milk, creamed cottage cheese, and ice cream. These products should be avoided or limited. Egg yolks are the highest source of dietary cholesterol available. All of the cholesterol in an egg is contained in the yolk. With these general guidelines in mind, we will now interpret some product labels. For most products that have a high cholesterol and/or high saturated fat content, there is usually a low cholesterol, low saturated fat substitute available. It will take you time to find substitution products that appeal to your sense of taste, but it can be done. Remember, dietary control is the key to conquering cholesterol, and that begins with awareness of what you eat.

LABELS

Reading food labels and understanding the information on them will help you conquer cholesterol and make wise food choices. There is a lot of information on a label, and it can be confusing. Food labels generally contain three types of information: 1. the ingredients, 2. calorie content, and 3. nutritional information. All of the information on the label will help you control your cholesterol. The nutritional information will give you the amount of fat a product contains and may also tell you the cholesterol content, although this is not presently required. The ideal nutritional information will list the total fat content in grams (per serving), the saturated and polyunsaturated fat content, as well as the milligrams (mg.) of cholesterol.

Unfortunately, the cholesterol information is listed voluntarily as it is not presently required. There is no difficulty interpreting the fat and cholesterol data if it is present. As already discussed, low cholesterol content and using unsaturated fat products instead of saturated fat products are best for controlling your cholesterol level. Some labels do not include all of the nutritional information. When partial information is supplied, it will require you to investigate the label further. If the cholesterol content and/or the breakdown of saturated and unsaturated fat is not present, you must examine the ingredient part of the label.

The nutritional information for cholesterol is listed in milligrams (mg.). Remember, your total daily intake of cholesterol should be 250-300 mg. or less per day. All of the nutritional information is given for a specific serving size. If you use more than the listed serving portion you must multiply the information, and if you use less, you must divide the nutritional information to accurately reflect your intake. For example, if you use a mayonnaise that contains 20 mg. of cholesterol per tablespoon and you use two tablespoons, you are ingesting (2 × 20 = 40) 40 mg. of cholesterol.

The ingredient portion of the label lists from highest content to lowest content. That is, the first ingredient is present in the largest amount, and the last ingredient is present in the least amount. That means that if a margarine product lists liquid corn oil, partially hydrogenated corn oil, and water as its ingredients, the product contains mostly liquid corn oil. Partially hydrogenated corn oil is the second most prevalent ingredient and water is the least. It is best for the unsaturated fats to be present in the largest quantity. Saturated and hydrogenated fats should not be present at all, but, if present, they should be in small quantity. As unsaturated fats are better than saturated fats, so are partially hydrogenated fats better than hydrogenated fats. By knowing the "good" ingredients from the "bad", you can make wise cholesterol choices with limited nutritional information provided on the label.

The calorie content is useful to help obtain and maintain ideal body weight. (Obtaining and maintaining ideal body weight is discussed in detail in Chapter 8.) To take control of cholesterol and heart disease, you will need to examine all of the information provided on the label. A little practice makes this seemingly difficult task much easier than you might presently suspect.

Let's start with how to interpret the information by examining two sample product labels. After reviewing these labels, we will compare three labels for similar foods which have different cholesterol and fat content or different polyunsaturated:saturated fat ratios. This exercise will help prepare you for making wise food choices to control cholesterol.

SAMPLE LABEL #1

Campbell Chicken Noodle Soup

Serving Size	4 oz. condensed
	8 oz. prepared
Calories	70
Protein	3 gm.
Carbohydrates	9 gm. (total)
	[1 simple, 8 complex]
Fat	3 gm.
Sodium	840 mg./serving

Ingredients: Chicken stock, enriched egg noodles, chicken meat, water, salt, celery, potato starch, carrots, margarine, yeast extract and hydrolyzed vegetable protein, chicken fat, dehydrated onions, monosodium glutamate, natural flavorings, and dehydrated garlic

As you begin your examination of this label, you will see that in the nutritional information provided there is no breakdown of unsaturated to saturated fat, and there is no cholesterol content in milligrams. You know that this product contains a total of 3 grams of fat. It will be necessary to read the list of ingredients and make your evaluation of the type of fat based on this. The first ingredient listed in chicken stock. You know that chicken is a source of low cholesterol. (Chicken meat, which is the third ingredient, is also a low cholesterol food.) The next most prevalent ingredient is enriched egg noodles. Many noodles contain whole eggs or egg yolks and are usually listed as egg noodle somewhere on the label. Noodles are enriched when the flour has vitamins added. Knowing this piece of information tells you that Campbell's Chicken Noodle Soup probably contains cholesterol from egg yolks. Salt, celery, potato starch, and carrots are all cholesterol free. The vegetable ingredients are polyunsaturates and would be recommended as a "good" food choice. Margarine is used, *not* butter, so once again this is consistent with a low-cholesterol selection. Chicken fat is listed as an ingredient. Although chicken fat does not contain 29% saturated fat, it is listed as one of the last ingredients and, therefore, is present in a smaller quantity than the vegetable fat (margarine) listed. None of the other listed ingredients are made from an animal source or palm and/ or coconut. If you use the two rules for identifying food which contained saturated fats, you will determine that saturated fat is not contained in the remaining ingredients. You now need to think about the polyunsaturated to saturated fat ratio. You may have questioned whether or not the hydrolyzed vegetable protein was a saturated fat because the word hydrolyzed was used. In Chapter 2 we discussed the fact that vegetable fats that are hydrogenated are utilized by the body like a saturated fat as opposed to polyunsaturated. In other words, hydrogenated vegetable fats will raise your cholesterol level. This product, however, does not contain *hydrogenated fat* but *hydrolyzed protein*. Hydrolyzed protein does not elevate the blood cholesterol level.

Now, put all of the information together that you have obtained from reading this label. Most of the fat content is from chicken, which is a better meat source than beef or pork. The remaining fat source would be from the margarine, which is vegetable and is a polyunsaturated fat. But remember that there is cholesterol contained in this product due to the eggs used in the noodles which is the second most prevalent ingredient in this product. The maximum daily cholesterol intake should not exceed 250–

300 mg./day. You have to approximate cholesterol content since it is not specifically listed on the label. By looking in cholesterol content tables, you can approximate that a serving of enriched egg noodles contains about 50 mg. of cholesterol. If you consider the cholesterol content of this product in your daily allowance, this could be a good food choice for you. Ideally, the same soup would be better for you without egg noodles.

SAMPLE LABEL #2

Jif Creamy Peanut Butter

Serving Size: 2 Tablespoons

Calories: 190

Protein: 9 gm.

Carbohydrates: 6 gm.

Fat: 16 gm.

Polyunsaturated: 5 gm.

Saturated: 3 gm.

Cholesterol: 0 mg.

Ingredients: roasted peanuts, sugar, hardened vegetable oil, salt, molasses, mono and diglycerides

This label provides all of the information concerning the amounts of polyunsaturated and saturated fats present. In addition, cholesterol content is included in the nutritional portion of the label. When all of this information is provided, it makes the job of interpreting the label much easier. The first thing you want to consider is: Does this product contain cholesterol? The answer is no. You can see that this is clearly demonstrated in the nutritional information. But even if the label did not contain the cholesterol content of this product, you could examine the ingredients. In doing that, you find that there are no animal or dairy products present. This would indicate to you that there is no cholesterol contained in this peanut butter. After determining if cholesterol is present in the product, you then must determine the polyunsaturated-:saturated fat ratio. Once again this label actually tells you that there are 5 gm. of polyunsaturated and 3 gm. saturated fat contained in the product. This product contains more unsaturated than saturated fat. This is an example in which the total grams of fat are listed as 16 and combined total of polyunsaturated and saturated fat is 8 grams. Remember, in Chapter 3 you learned that peanuts and peanut oil are monounsaturates. The remaining 8 grams of fat in this product are monounsaturated.

Interpreting the Label

It is best to get into the habit of reading food labels in the grocery before you buy. If you read labels after the product is purchased, chances are you will eat the food even though you determine that it is high in cholesterol and/or saturated fat. To repeat, there are three types of information on food labels: the nutritional content, calorie content, and ingredient information. Compare various food products to make the best low cholesterol, low saturated fat choice. There are many products that you think are similar until you examine the label. Here are some tips for comparing and making the right choice for your heart.

Under the nutritional information the label will list the serving size. All of the remaining information given is dependent on the serving size, so pay attention and adjust according to your portions. Nutritional information includes the calories, protein, and carbohydrate and fat content. As we have discussed in the previous section, some labels will distinguish between the amount of saturated and polyunsaturated fats, while others will list only a total fat content. If the label lists only the total fat content, you will then have to rely on the list of ingredients to decide if the product contains more saturated or unsaturated fats. Some food labels now contain the cholesterol content of the food. If the package has that information, it will be listed under the fat content.

Here are examples of three food labels. The first contains only the total fat content, the second example gives the saturated: polyunsaturated breakdown, and the third gives the saturated/polyunsaturated information plus the cholesterol content.

BRIGHT DAY SALAD DRESSING
  Serving Size: 1 Tablespoon
  Calories: 60
  Protein: 0 gm.
  Carbohydrates: 2 gm.
  Fat: 6 gm.
  Cholesterol: 0 mg.

IMITATION MAYONNAISE
  Serving Size: 1 Tablespoon
  Calories: 40
  Protein: 0 gm.
  Carbohydrate: 1 gm.
  Fat: 4 gm.
     Polyunsaturated: 3 gm.
     Saturated: 1 gm.

REAL MAYONNAISE
Serving Size: 1 Tablespoon
Calories: 100
Protein: 0 gm.
Carbohydrates: 0 gm.
Fat: 11 gm.
  Polyunsaturated: 7 gm.
  Saturated: 2 gm.
Cholesterol: 100 mg.

In the last example notice that the total fat content is 11 grams, yet the total of the polyunsaturated (7 gm.) and saturated (2 gm.) is only 9 grams. What happened to the other 2 grams? Most labeling tends to ignore the monounsaturated fat content. Thus the "missing" two grams are monounsaturated. If you "see" missing grams of fat on a label, you can assume that they are due to monounsaturated fats, which may also help lower your blood cholesterol. Monounsaturated fats also contribute 9 calories per gram just like any other fat source.

By taking the time to examine the package label you will see that these three products that look and taste similar are not the same when it comes to the fat content. Look at the nutritional information that is provided on these labels, and you will see the choice for a healthy heart becomes clearer.

Now let's check the ingredients of the product. The ingredients are listed from the highest to the lowest total weight content. When looking at a food product, you will have to keep in mind what food sources provide saturated fat (foods of animal origin, dairy products, palm and coconut oils) and the sources of polyunsaturated fats (vegetable products with the exception of palm and coconut). Remember, you want to examine foods for a polyunsaturated:saturated fat ratio of at least 2:1. That is, they should contain twice as many polyunsaturated fats as saturated fats. Let's now examine the ingredients of these three products.

BRIGHT DAY SALAD DRESSING

Soybean oil, distilled vinegar, water, cider vinegar, corn syrup, egg whites, food starch, modified sugar, salt, mustard flour, spice, oleo resins, paprika, calcium disodium

IMITATION MAYONNAISE

Water, soybean oil, food starch, vinegar, sugar, salt, lemon juice, egg yolks, mustard flour, xanthum gum

REAL MAYONNAISE

Soybean oil, vinegar, whole eggs, egg yolks, water, salt, sweeteners

In examining the three labels, you should first determine their relative cholesterol content and then their polyunsaturated:saturated fat ratio. If the cholesterol content is equal, then the best choice would be the food with the highest polyunsaturated:saturated fat ratio. If the cholesterol content is not equal, then the best choice is the product containing the lowest cholesterol. That is assuming that the total fat content as well as the polyunsaturated:saturated (P:S) ratio are not *extremely* different. You should always try to keep the cholesterol content as low as possible and the P:S ratio as high as possible in the foods you eat.

Reviewing the mayonnaise labels reveals that the Real Mayonnaise contains 100 mg. of cholesterol per tablespoon. This means your total daily maximum cholesterol allowance is contained in 2 ¹/₂ to 3 tablespoons. This cholesterol content is quite high. If you look at the list of ingredients, you will see the reason for the high cholesterol content. The third and fourth ingredients are whole eggs and egg yolks, both high in cholesterol. The Bright Days Salad Dressing and the Imitation Mayonnaise do not list cholesterol content in the nutritional information. But examining the list of ingredients will help you determine the relative cholesterol content. The Imitation Mayonnaise lists egg yolks as the eighth ingredient; whereas, the Bright Days Salad Dressing lists only egg whites as the sixth ingredient. As you have learned, all of the cholesterol in an egg is contained in the yolk. Therefore, Imitation Mayonnaise must have a higher cholesterol content than Bright Days Salad Dressing. In the same way, Imitation Mayonnaise would be expected to have a lower cholesterol content than Real Mayonnaise, which contains whole eggs and egg yolks as the third and fourth most prevalent ingredients. By examining the ingredients, we know that Real Mayonnaise is the highest in cholesterol and Bright Days Salad Dressing is the lowest, with Imitation Mayonnaise between the two. Comparing the fat content of the two lowest cholesterol products, we find 6 gm./tablespoon for the Bright Days Salad Dressing versus 4 gm./tablespoon for Imitation. The fat content for the Imitation Mayonnaise has a P:S ratio of 3. The 6 grams of fat in Bright Days Salad Dressing is not broken down into polyunsaturated/saturated fat. Now look back at the list of ingredients. The major fat ingredient of Bright Days Salad Dressing is soybean oil, which has a good P:S ratio. As a matter of fact, the major fat ingredient in Imitation

Mayonnaise is also soybean oil. You would thus expect the P:S ratio of Bright Days Salad Dressing to not only be "good" but to be similar to Imitation Mayonnaise. You can then conclude that, even though Bright Days Salad Dressing has more total fat (6 grams) than Imitation Mayonnaise (4 grams), it is the best cholesterol choice. This is based on the fact that it has the lowest cholesterol content of the three choices and a similar P:S ratio as the next best choice, Imitation Mayonnaise. Bright Days Salad Dressing would still be the best choice if the P:S ratio is 2:1 since it contains no cholesterol.

Practice, Practice, Practice

Reading labels may seem a bit frustrating and time consuming if you do not presently look at food labels critically. But if you keep reading and practicing, it will soon become second nature to you. Since anything becomes easier with some practice, the next few pages are samples of actual food labels for you to interpret and compare. At the end of the samples there are questions to see if you made the best choice available. There are also comments about how to arrive at the best choice. Don't worry; time and practice will make it all easy for you to be the wise shopper your heart deserves. If you take the time now to examine what you eat, you will have the time later to enjoy good health.

The following are sample product labels. These are included in this chapter to give you some practice in interpretation. Interpret the labels by asking yourself: Does this product contain cholesterol? What is the polyunsaturated:saturated fat ratio? Remember, the ideal P:S ratio should be 2:1 or greater.

RAGU SPAGHETTI SAUCE

Serving Size: 4 oz.

Calories: 80

Protein: 2 gm.

Carbohydrates: 11 gm.

Fat: 3 gm.

Cholesterol: 0 mg. (0 mg./100 gm)

Ingredients: tomatoes, soybean oil, salt, corn syrup, dried onions, Romano cheese made from cows' milk, olive oil, spices, garlic powder

When you examine the label for the Ragu Spaghetti Sauce, you see that the cholesterol content has been provided for you, but not the polyunsaturated and saturated fat content. The first consideration—Does this product contain cholesterol?—is clearly provided for you. The answer is no. You can now address the question—Is there a 2:1 ratio of polyunsaturated to saturated fat? This is not specifically stated on the label, so you will have to use the ingredient list to analyze the 3 grams of fat. Tomatoes are vegetables, so they do not contain saturated fats. Soybean oil is a polyunsaturated fat. It is better to have a fat in the liquid form (as it is in this product) than partially or completely hydrogenated. Salt, corn syrup, and dried onions are not considerations in regard to cholesterol and fat content. Romano cheese made from cows' milk will have some butterfat contained in it. Olive oil is one of the monounsaturated fats and, therefore, not a factor in determining P:S ratio. The two remaining ingredients— spices and garlic powder—do not contain fats. In examining this label you find that most of the 3 gm. will be either polyunsaturated (soybean oil) or monounsaturated (olive oil) with a small portion of the Romano cheese containing butterfat from the milk. This product would be a wise low cholesterol, low saturated fat food choice.

KRAFT MACARONI AND CHEESE DINNER

Serving Size: ¹/₄ Box or ³/₄ Cup Prepared*

	Box	Prepared
Calories:	190	290
Protein:	9 gm.	9 gm.
Carbohydrates:	36 gm.	34 gm.
Fat:	2 gm.	13 gm.

Ingredients: enriched macaroni, cheese sauce (whey, dehydrated cheese), [granular cheddar, (milk, cheese cultures, salt, enzymes)], whey, protein concentrate, skim milk, salt, buttermilk, sodium tripolyphosphate, sodium phosphate, citric acid, yellow no. 5 color, artificial color, lactic acid

The practice label for the Kraft Macaroni and Cheese Dinner does not give all of the nutritional information in regard to unsaturated and saturated fat content or cholesterol. You, therefore, have to use the ingredient portion of the label. This product contains enriched macaroni, cheese, milk, skim milk, and butter milk. You can deduce that at least some cholesterol is present, from the eggs in the macaroni and from the milk and cheese. The fat that is contained in this product is all saturated fat since it is all from animal sources. There are no polyunsaturated vegetable fats present in the list of ingredients. You could increase or decrease the amount of butterfat contained in this prepared product depending upon whether you used whole or skim milk in the preparation. The package direc-

---

* Package directions state to add margarine and milk to box contents.

tions do not specifically state if whole or skim milk should be used. That makes it impossible to accurately utilize the information on the box about prepared nutritional information.

PEPPERIDGE FARM GOLDFISH THINS CHEESE CRACKERS

Serving Size: 4 crackers

Calories: 70

Protein: 1 gm.

Carbohydrates: 8 gm.

Fat: 3 gm.

Ingredients: unbleached flour, modified food starch, coconut oil, partially hydrogenated vegetable shortening (soybean/cottonseed or coconut), farina, cheddar cheese, salt, dehydrated processed cheddar cheese, Parmesan, leavening agents, baking soda, cream of tartar, sugar, yeast, onion powder, protase

We have included the Pepperidge Farms Goldfish Thins Cheese Crackers as a practice label for several reasons. Most nutritional labeling for crackers and cracker products consists of only the ingredient list. You will be required to deduce the approximate amount and type of fat contained in the product. You will also have to determine from the ingredient list if there is cholesterol contained in the product. Many people who are trying to adopt a nutritious and healthful way of eating choose crackers as a snack food. But just how low in saturated fat and cholesterol are snack crackers? The ingredient list contains several sources of saturated fat. Coconut oil (a saturated fat) is the third ingredient listed. The fourth most prevalent ingredient is hydrogenated vegetable shortening. Once again this is a saturated fat. The type of vegetable shortening that may be used in this product is either soybean/cottonseed or coconut. In addition to the coconut oil and partially hydrogenated shortening, dairy fats are contained in the form of cheddar cheese, dehydrated cheddar cheese, and Parmesan. In analyzing this label we would conclude that saturated fats are contained in these crackers. Additionally, there is no evidence of polyunsaturated fat in the crackers. This item obviously does not meet the recommendation of polyunsaturated to saturated fat ratio of 2:1. By reviewing this ingredient list you can conclude that this is not a good low saturated fat food.

KELLOGG'S CORN FLAKES

Serving Size: 1 oz. (about 1 cup with $1/2$ cup skim milk)

	Cereal	With Skim Milk
Calories:	110	150*
Protein:	2 gm.	6 gm.
Carbohydrates:	25 gm.	31 gm.
Fat:	0 gm.	0 gm.*
Cholesterol:	0 mg.	0 mg.*

Ingredients: corn, sugar, salt, malt flavoring, corn syrup

* Whole milk supplies an additional 30 calories, 4 gm. fat, and 15 mg. cholesterol.

The sample label for Kellogg's Corn Flakes shows that there is no fat and no cholesterol contained in this product. The dry cereal is a good food choice. The label further informs the consumer that whole milk will add 4 grams of fat and 15 mg. of cholesterol, while skim milk adds no fat and no cholesterol. The fat from milk products is a saturated fat. There are no polyunsaturated fats contained to "balance" this food with a good P:S ratio. Once again, you can see that the use of skim milk over whole or 2% milk is the best low cholesterol choice.

These samples have given you an opportunity to practice interpreting labels. Get into the habit of reviewing product labels before you buy, so that you will have low cholesterol, low-fat foods in your home. Look at all parts of the label. As you have seen, labels differ in the amount and type of information they provide. Examine the ingredient list and continue to look for all sources of fat and cholesterol in products. Fat should be identified as polyunsaturated, saturated, and monounsaturated. Remember, the polyunsaturated to saturated fat ratio should be at least 2:1. Label interpretation will get easier with practice, and it is well worth the time it takes to bring good food home to increase your chances of maintaining a healthy heart.

Here are two frozen food products that you might consider if you want an Italian dinner. Pick the best low cholesterol, low saturated fat choice.

RONZONI PASTA PRIMAVERA

Serving Size: 10 oz.

Calories: 340

Protein: 12 gm.

Carbohydrates: 39 gm.

Fat: 15 gm.

Ingredients: enriched macaroni, water, broccoli, carrots, snow peas, mushrooms, Parmesan cheese, butter, corn starch, chicken broth, walnut oil, garlic, soybean oil, water, hydrolyzed vegetable protein, salt, sugar, spices, onion powder, dry yeast

RONZONI FETTUCCINE ALFREDO

Serving Size: 10 oz.

Calories: 420

Protein: 16 gm.

Carbohydrate: 33 gm.

Fat: 25 gm.

Ingredients: enriched egg noodles, water, sour cream, Parmesan cheese, butter, cornstarch, salt, spices

Is one of these products a better low-fat choice? If you answer yes, which one and why? You can see that the labels list the total fat content only. The polyunsaturated fat, saturated fat, and cholesterol content are not listed. Pasta Primavera contains a total of 15 gm. of fat while the Fettuccine Alfredo contains 25 gm. of fat. You must then examine the ingredients to identify the source of cholesterol and fats. Pasta Primavera contains enriched macaroni, Parmesan cheese, butter, chicken broth, walnut oil, and soybean oil. These ingredients are all sources of fat. Once you have identified the fat sources, you must then categorize them as polyunsaturated or saturated. The enriched macaroni, Parmesan cheese, butter, and chicken broth would all contain some cholesterol and/or saturated fats. There would be very little cholesterol in the chicken broth, and according to the list of ingredients, there is not much broth contained in this product. Therefore, cholesterol content from this ingredient is minimal. Walnut oil and soybean oil are both polyunsaturated fats. Walnut oil also contains omega-3 fatty acids. The Fettuccine Alfredo contains enriched egg noodles, sour cream, Parmesan cheese, and butter. All of these ingredients are saturated fats, and the eggs in the enriched noodles contain cholesterol. There are no polyunsaturated fats contained in the Fettuccine Alfredo. All 25 grams of fat contained in this product are saturated. The 15 grams of fat contained in the Pasta Primavera are a combination of polyunsaturated and saturated. Of the 15 grams more are saturated, but there are some polyunsaturated fat. While it would probably not meet the 2:1 P:S ratio, it is better than the Fettuccine Alfredo as a low-fat choice. The Fettuccine Alfredo probably also contains more cholesterol than does the Pasta Primavera. The overall winner in these two examples would be the Pasta Primavera. It contains less overall fat content. It has both polyunsaturated and saturated fat, and less cholesterol. In reality, neither pasta product would be a wise low-fat, low cholesterol choice. A substitute product should be found, or you should make the pasta of your choice with low-fat substitutes (see Chapter 11).

FOODS HIGH IN CHOLESTEROL

Liver	Kidneys
Sweetbreads	Brains
Heart	Chitterlings
Gizzard	Egg Yolk

FOODS MODERATELY HIGH IN CHOLESTEROL

Shrimp

Lobster

Sardines

Skin of Chicken and Turkey

You can make many low cholesterol, low saturated fat food choices to substitute for those foods that promote heart disease. Following are some samples of similar products. Those listed in Column I are high in cholesterol and/or saturated fats while those in Column II are wise substitutions.

COLUMN I	COLUMN II
Whole Milk =	.5% Milk =
3.5% Butterfat	0.5% Butterfat
1 cup	1 cup
150 calories	90 calories
8 gm. fat	1 gm. fat
34 mg. cholesterol	5 mg. cholesterol
Butter =	Margarine =
1 tablespoon	1 tablespoon
12 gm. fat	12 gm. fat
35 mg. cholesterol	0 mg. cholesterol
Whole Egg =	Egg Beaters =
1 egg	1 serving
80 calories	35 calories
6 gm. fat	2 gm. fat
275 mg. cholesterol	0 mg. cholesterol
Flavored Yogurt =	Plain Yogurt =
1 cup (8 oz.)	1 cup (8 oz.)
230 calories	150 calories
7 gm. fat	4 gm. fat
17 mg. cholesterol	6 mg. cholesterol
Creamed Cottage Cheese =	Low Fat Cottage Cheese =
1 cup (8 oz.)	1 cup (8 oz.)
260 calories	170 calories
10 gm. fat	1 gm. fat
48 mg. cholesterol	13 mg. cholesterol

(Continued on next page)

COLUMN I	COLUMN II
Ice cream =	Ice Milk (no palm or coconut oil) Vanilla flavored =
1 cup (8 oz.)	1 cup (8 oz.)
255 calories	100 calories
9 gm. fat	2 gm. fat
35 mg. cholesterol	10 mg. cholesterol

CHOLESTEROL CONTENT OF MEAT AND MEAT PRODUCTS

Food	Serving Size	Cholesterol
Fish (lean)	3 oz.	63 mg.
Chicken (skinless)	3 oz.	74 mg.
Turkey (skinless)	3 oz.	74 mg.
Cold Cuts	3 oz.	82 mg.
Beef Prime Rib	3 oz.	85 mg.
Hamburger (25% fat)	3 oz.	85 mg.
Veal Cutlet	3 oz.	86 mg.

6 Checking Lipid Levels

To determine your cholesterol level requires having a blood test performed. A screening cholesterol test may be performed either fasting or nonfasting. The data show that total cholesterol levels are equally reliable in the fasting or nonfasting state. If a triglyceride level and the HDL cholesterol are being measured, then the blood specimen should be drawn after you have been fasting for a minimum of twelve hours. Most cholesterol levels are checked by having blood drawn from a vein (usually in the arm). The blood that is drawn can be checked for triglycerides and total cholesterol, as well as HDL, the good cholesterol component. The LDL can not be directly measured in the blood. However, there is a way to calculate the amount of LDL cholesterol by knowing the total cholesterol, triglycerides, and HDL. This is sometimes referred to as an indirect measurement, because it is derived indirectly from the other known information. The formula for calculating the LDL cholesterol is:

LDL = Total Cholesterol − Triglycerides ÷ 5 − HDL

For example, if your cholesterol = 220, HDL = 45,
and triglycerides = 125, your LDL cholesterol would be

$$220(C) - 125(Tri) \div 5 - 45 (HDL) =$$
$$220 - 25 - 45 = 150 (LDL)$$

Cholesterol is measured in milligrams (mg.) in $^1/_{10}$ liter
of blood (dL). For example, if your cholesterol level was
reported to be 180 mg./dL, that would mean that every
$^1/_{10}$ liter of your blood contains 180 mg. of cholesterol.
Mg./dL is the standard unit of cholesterol measurement in
the U.S., but levels are generally spoken about (impre-
cisely) without the units or sometimes just as mgs. The
recommendation from the National Institutes of Health
(NIH) and the American Heart Association (AHA) is to
reduce blood cholesterol to 200 mg./dL or less for all
adults. The average blood cholesterol for Americans
between the ages of 35 and 60 years was 211 mg./dL in
1984. That is a decrease from the average of 250 mg./dL in
1978. While these numbers show us that the trend in the
United States is toward lower cholesterol levels, it is
important to realize that the average cholesterol level of
men who had a heart attack was 225 mg./dL. This is one
of the reasons that the recommendation for the total cholesterol level is 200 mg./dL or less for all Americans over
the age of two. There is a distinct difference between the
"normal" level and the "recommended" level of blood
cholesterol. The meaning of "normal" cholesterol level is
based on the cholesterol level of a large number of Americans. A "mean value" and "standard deviation" are calculated from these values and the "normal levels" are thus
determined. Unfortunately, because the American diet is
high in cholesterol and saturated fats, the "normal levels"
were determined to be quite high. The "recommended
levels" are based on scientific studies which have shown at
what level the risk of cardiovascular disease increases.
Thus, the recommended levels are much lower than the
previously accepted normal levels. For this reason the

American Heart Association and the NIH have re-evaluated the normal total cholesterol level for American adults. The current recommended normal of 200 mg./dL is to try to minimize the risk for heart disease. *The first attempts at lowering cholesterol level to achieve the recommended value should always be dietary modifications.* This is done by reducing the total cholesterol and saturated fat intake. The total intake of fats should be limited to 30%, with less than 10% from saturated fats, up to 10% from polyunsaturated and 10-15% monounsaturated fats. The maximum daily cholesterol intake should be 250-300 mgs. If this diet is not successful in reaching the desired cholesterol level, a stricter diet containing less cholesterol and fat should be instituted. In addition, other dietary changes, such as decreasing calorie intake to obtain ideal body weight, should be employed. This and other ideas will be discussed in later chapters.

Everyone is encouraged to have his/her blood cholesterol level checked. You should be as aware of your cholesterol level as you are of your blood pressure. If the total cholesterol level is within the recommended limits (less than 200 mg./dL) and there are no other risk factors for heart disease present, the cholesterol can be checked every five years. If the total cholesterol is borderline high at 200-239 mg./dL, there is a moderately increased risk of developing heart disease. At this cholesterol range, dietary modification should be made and the cholesterol level rechecked within one year. However, if there is coronary artery disease or two risk factors present, a lipid profile should be obtained. These risk factors include hypertension, smoking, family history of heart disease, male, obesity, diabetes, history of peripheral vascular disease, or a low HDL cholesterol. Treatment and repeat cholesterol determinations would be based on the LDL cholesterol levels. (See Chapter 9 for more specific information.) If the cholesterol level is 240 mg./dL or above, the individual is considered to be in the high-risk category for developing coronary heart disease. A lipid profile should be obtained to help your personal physician prescribe dietary modifications and any necessary medication therapy. This will be at the discretion of your physician and will depend on the individual cholesterol level and overall risk factors. If a person is in the high-risk category, the cholesterol level should be repeated to confirm the abnormal results. The cholesterol level should then be repeated as necessary to monitor dietary and/or medication effects. This can be done as frequently as once a month or, typically, every two to four months, until the desired levels are obtained. Cholesterol monitoring can then be done on a yearly basis or more frequently if your physician feels it is appropriate. Because of the increased demands to have cholesterol levels performed quickly, easily, and above all accurately, new techniques are being developed. Several machines are currently available which can determine a cholesterol level within minutes from blood obtained by a simple finger stick. This technique allows for mass screening of cholesterol in doctors' offices, work settings, clinics, and health fairs. However, only total cholesterol and triglycerides are generally available by this technique. HDL cholesterol is not always available, depending on the type of machine used. Anyone with an elevated total cholesterol or abnormally high triglycerides should have a fasting specimen obtained for HDL cholesterol as well as for triglycerides.

BLOOD CHOLESTEROL LEVELS

Less than 200 mg./dL   Desirable

200-239 mg./dL   Borderline–High

Greater than or
equal to 240 mg./dL   High

TRIGLYCERIDES

Triglycerides are another type of lipid in the blood. The role of triglycerides in the development and progression of atherosclerosis is currently not well defined. Medically there is little known about triglycerides. What is known, however, is that elevation of the triglyceride level is frequently associated with cholesterol elevation. Triglycerides are not generally an independent factor in cardiovascular disease, but rather a predictor that other risk factors may be present. For instance, elevation of triglycerides is seen in association with obesity, diabetes, thyroid disease, and alcohol consumption, all of which increase the risk of cardiovascular disease. There is also some evidence that triglyceride levels increase with cigarette smoking and a sedentary lifestyle. Once again, both of these are risk factors for cardiovascular disease. Triglyceride elevation, therefore, may signal other associated risk factors or be part of a larger problem of elevated total cholesterol. An elevated triglyceride level is an independent risk factor in women. Due to the fact that elevated triglyceride levels are associated with additional risks for coronary artery disease in men, and as an independent risk in women, the blood triglyceride level should be checked and monitored. The NIH consensus panel report recommended that triglycerides between 250 and 500 mg./dL should be used as a marker to carefully evaluate for other risk factors. The consensus panel further recommended that anyone with a triglyceride level above 500 mg./dL should be treated with diet and drug therapy. (See Chapter 9 for drug therapy.)

The definitive answers to the role of triglycerides in the development and progression of atherosclerosis is not clear. But since there is an association between triglyceride elevation and cardiovascular disease, it is best to control the triglyceride blood level as well as the cholesterol level.

Types of Hypercholesterolemia

As you remember from Chapter 2, the term lipid refers to any of the fats in the blood. The term *hyperlipidemia* simply means that one of the fats in the blood is elevated, either cholesterol or triglycerides. The term *hypercholesterolemia* specifically means that the blood cholesterol level is elevated above the recommended levels. (The prefix "hyper" means increased or above normal.) As you have learned in the first part of this chapter, blood tests can directly measure the total cholesterol level, as well as HDL and triglycerides. From this information, the LDL cholesterol level can be calculated. When each category or specific lipid is analyzed, the exact cause for the high lipid level (hyperlipidemia) can be appreciated. Depending upon which component of the lipid profile is elevated, a specific name or type is given to that particular pattern of elevation. The simplified table that follows defines the types of hyperlipidemias and their arbitrary definitions. Type II is the most prevalent form of hypercholesterolemia found in the United States. Type II is divided into two categories, Type IIa and Type IIb.

Type IIa means that the total blood cholesterol is elevated and the triglycerides are normal. An elevation in the LDL cholesterol component is what causes an elevation in the total cholesterol. In other words, the person said to have Type IIa hyperlipidemia has so much of the LDL, or bad cholesterol, that the total cholesterol is elevated. Type IIb hypercholesterolemia means that there is an elevation in the triglycerides as well as total cholesterol. The total cholesterol elevation is due to increased levels of LDL cholesterol and increased triglyceride levels. If we rearrange the formula previously used to calculate LDL, we see that:

Total Cholesterol = LDL + HDL + triglycerides ÷ 5

Therefore, an elevated triglyceride level will increase the measured total cholesterol blood level without necessarily increasing LDL level. Type IIa and IIb are the two most prevalent kinds of hypercholesterolemia. Both will respond to dietary management. Reducing the amount of saturated fats and cholesterol is the first step in the management of hypercholesterolemia. Drugs are never a substitute for dietary control. There are studies that show a diet high in saturated fats may actually override the effects of drugs used to lower cholesterol levels. In keeping with this same line of thinking, the amount of drug therapy necessary to control elevated cholesterol may be reduced with the addition of a low-fat, low cholesterol diet.

The additional categories of hyperlipidemia are Type I, Type III, Type IV, and Type V. These types are found much less commonly in the general population than Type II, and will not be discussed. The classifications were originally used for laboratory convenience only and have no relationship to the cause of the problem. Regardless of the specific type of hyperlipidemia you may have, it is important to remember that dietary control of saturated fats and cholesterol is the cornerstone to therapy. Without dietary modifications, it is impossible to effectively control any type of hyperlipidemia.

	Cholesterol	Triglycerides	LDL	HDL
Type I	↑	↑↑↑	↓↓	↓↓
Type IIa	↑↑	—	↑↑	—
Type IIb	↑↑	↑	↑↑	↓
Type III	↑↑	↑↑	—	↓
Type IV	↑	↑↑	—	↓
Type V	↑↑	↑↑↑	↓	↓↓

↑ Small Increase   ↓ Small Decrease
↑↑ Moderate Increase   ↓↓ Moderate Decrease
↑↑↑ Large Increase   ↓↓↓ Large Decrease
— Normal

FACTORS THAT AFFECT BLOOD CHOLESTEROL LEVELS

In addition to the food you eat, several other factors will affect your blood cholesterol level. These include your weight, how much you exercise, smoking, stress level, the amount of fiber and sugar in your diet, certain diseases, and some side effects of certain medications, especially medicines used to control high blood pressure. Also, an inherited genetic defect which affects the liver's ability to process cholesterol is found in about 1 in 500 people with elevated blood cholesterol levels. Obviously, other than an inherited genetic defect, most of these factors which affect cholesterol can be modified in a favorable manner.

The next chapter (Chapter 7) deals briefly with those diseases which have the most effect on the cholesterol level, as well as the medications that most commonly affect cholesterol as an undesirable side effect. In addition, fiber in the diet is discussed. These factors are less common and usually have less overall effect on the cholesterol blood level than does weight control, exercise, and smoking. Because of their importance, weight control, exercise, and smoking are discussed in more detail in Chapter 8.

7

Other Factors That Affect Lipids

There are a group of recognized factors, other than diet and genetic makeup, that can affect your blood cholesterol levels. Some of these factors are harmful and may raise the LDL cholesterol, whereas others, such as fiber, may actually help reduce cholesterol levels. First we will discuss the factors that can raise the blood cholesterol level.

Cholesterol levels can increase as a result of some ailments such as hypothyroidism, diabetes, and some types of liver and kidney disease. This elevation of cholesterol is considered "secondary" because it happens as a result of a "primary" disease or problem. The treatment of choice of these secondary problems is to treat the underlying primary disease. It is important to re-emphasize at this point, that even if the cause of your elevated cholesterol is secondary to another problem, a low cholesterol, low saturated fat diet is usually still recommended. This goes back to the fact that the normal American diet is too high in cholesterol and saturated fat.

In addition to the above diseases, secondary elevation of blood cholesterol level can occur when taking certain medications. The following are some medications that have been extensively studied and proven to elevate cholesterol levels. Anabolic steroids and progesterones, particularly those which do not contain estrogens, are two medications that have been shown to elevate LDL cholesterol levels and drastically reduce HDL cholesterol. If these medications are necessary for the treatment of a disease or medical condition, they should be regulated by a physician. The cholesterol levels will then be checked during the course of drug therapy. These medications become particularly dangerous when individuals take them without the recommendation and follow up of a physician. Anabolic steroids that are taken without supervision by athletes and body builders may have very serious consequences by possibly accelerating atherosclerosis, which can lead to heart attack or stroke. Anabolic steroids have been shown to reduce the HDL cholesterol by as much as 10% to 70%. Studies of the effects of progesterones show a decrease in HDL cholesterol of 5% to 15%.

Some medications that are used in the treatment of hypertension raise total cholesterol. They do this by raising the LDL cholesterol and triglycerides while decreasing the beneficial HDL cholesterol. Medications that are used in the treatment of hypertension must be carefully regulated by a physician. Persons taking these medications should not discontinue or reduce the dosage without the consent of a physician. The possibility of suffering a stroke or heart attack from uncontrolled hypertension is high. The beneficial effects of controlling hypertension with certain medications must be weighed against their detrimental side effect of elevating the cholesterol level. Specifically, several diuretics (water pills) used to treat hypertension can elevate cholesterol levels. They raise LDL cholesterol levels and triglycerides as well as lower HDL cholesterol levels. Beta blockers are another type of antihypertensive medication that affect the cholesterol. Beta blockers elevate triglycerides and lower HDL cholesterol levels. The beta blockers usually have more effect on the blood cholesterol levels than the diuretics. Remember, medications are *not* to be discontinued or altered without the recommendation of your physician.

Diabetes is a risk factor, independent of elevated cholesterol, for coronary heart disease. In diabetes there is a change in the way fats are used by the body, with a tendency to have an increased serum triglyceride level. There are also alterations seen in the blood vessels of diabetics. Because of the high risk associated with diabetes, there are specific recommendations that have been written for this group of people. The recommendations from the NIH Cholesterol Adult Treatment Panel Report states that men with diabetes should lower their LDL cholesterol to less than 130 mg./dL and women to less than 160 mg./dL. If the woman has other risk factors for heart disease, the LDL should be reduced to 130 mg./dL. Some of these additional risk factors are hypertension, smoking, family history of heart disease, and personal history of angina or heart attack. The same dietary plan is recommended for diabetics as for the general population. (See Chapter 4.)

If you have hypothyroidism, obstructive liver disease, or kidney disease, you should talk with your physician about your cholesterol levels. Be aware that all of these conditions may affect your cholesterol. The specifics of your particular condition will dictate a course of treatment for you. Remember, the first step in lowering your cholesterol level is to follow the diet changes discussed in this book.

What is the role of fiber in reducing cholesterol levels? There are two types of fiber, insoluble and soluble. The insoluble fiber has no effect on cholesterol. This type of fiber is the indigestible carbohydrate found in an average diet. An example of an insoluble fiber is cellulose which is found in wheat bran and celery. Insoluble fiber adds bulk to the stool but does nothing to lower cholesterol levels. The second type of fiber is soluble and has been shown to lower cholesterol levels. This fiber is soluble (dissolves) in the intestine but is not absorbed. Some examples of soluble fiber are pectins, certain gums, and psyllium. Pectins are found in many fruits, and one of the beneficial gums is found in oats and beans. Psyllium is the ingredient in Metamucil that has been shown to reduce cholesterol. Studies have shown that eating 15 to 25 grams per day of soluble fiber may lower total cholesterol 5% to 15%.Other studies have shown that fiber is most effective when cholesterol levels are quite high and the diet is bad— that is, higher in fats and cholesterol than has been recommended. Oat bran and oatmeal have been quite popular. Gram for gram, oat bran is twice as effective in lowering cholesterol than oatmeal. There are two drawbacks to using fiber. The first is that generally large quantities of fiber must be consumed to be effective. The second drawback is that fiber is least effective when used in conjunction with a low fat, low cholesterol diet. Still, fiber may help lower cholesterol 5-15%. Some people have gastrointestinal irritability with large amounts of fiber, but it appears that with longterm use, the side effects decrease.

8 Take Control of Your Cholesterol

Chest pain, heart attack, and stroke can have a devastating effect on your life. Do you want these problems to be part of your future? If not, it is up to you to do *all* that you can to prevent them. In addition to lowering your LDL cholesterol and triglycerides and raising your HDL cholesterol, you may have to make other changes. But isn't life worth it? We have spent a large portion of this book telling you why controlling cholesterol is important. The best way to lower cholesterol is to reduce total fat intake and limit the amount of saturated fat and cholesterol in your diet. These, in fact, are the guidelines set by the American Heart Association. In addition, obtaining and maintaining ideal body weight, adhering to a program of regular exercise, stopping smoking, and taking lipid lowering medications as they have been prescribed by your physician also help to control your lipid levels. You have learned about cholesterol and fats from reading Chapters 1–7. Now we will discuss some of the other ways to help control your lipids.

OBTAINING AND MAINTAINING
IDEAL BODY WEIGHT

Appendix 4 contains a height and weight chart listing ideal body weights. This chart is based on your height, sex, and bone structure. The table categorizes according to small, medium, and large bone structure or frame. It is easy to determine into which category you fit. Categories are determined by the diameter of the bony part of your wrist. To make this measurement, circle your wrist with your thumb and index finger. Use the wrist of your dominant hand and the thumb and index finger of your nondominant hand to make the determination. For example, if you are right handed, place the thumb and index finger of your left hand around your right wrist. If your thumb and index finger do not meet you have a large bone frame. If the thumb and index finger just meet, you have a medium frame; and if they overlap, you have a small frame.

It is important to know your ideal body weight so that you can achieve a realistic goal. Your idea of your "ideal body weight" may be different from the chart prepared by Metropolitan Life. The table is based on reality, as opposed to the fantasy that some of us create for ourselves. Use the table with the height, sex, and bone structure variables to find your ideal weight. Notice also that the weights are given in a range rather than one single figure. Practically speaking, everyone has fluctuations in weight. Keep in mind the ideal weight range rather than one particular number. Weight control must be practical, and that means working within a range.

If you find you are in the range of your ideal weight, you need not work to obtain your ideal weight, but rather to maintain it. The same strategies that we will discuss for obtaining ideal weight can be used for maintenance once the ideal weight has been reached. The suggestions and ideas we recommend for weight and cholesterol control will work for a lifetime. This is not a "diet" you go on and off but rather a pleasant, practical approach to eating. One of the reasons that fad diets don't work is that they aren't realistic over the long haul. Who can eat tuna fish and lettuce everyday for the rest of his/her life?

To obtain and maintain your ideal body weight it will be necessary for you to examine your eating habits. Because that's what eating is—a habit. Most of the time we eat without thinking very much about it. It is this mindless eating that can cause overeating and habits that contribute to being overweight. The following are some suggestions that give you greater control over eating, as well as adding greater pleasure and satisfaction. Eating should be pleasurable, but to increase the pleasure you have to pay attention. This new awareness to eating will help with both cholesterol and weight control.

PAY ATTENTION TO YOUR BODY'S SIGNALS

We eat to give our body the nutrients and energy it needs. Food is fuel for the body. If we give it too much food, the body will store the additional food as fuel for future use. Fat is the body's means of storage. To obtain and maintain your ideal weight, you must balance your intake of food and the expenditure of energy. Your body will tell you when it needs nutrients and energy. Unfortunately, most of us have not been conditioned to pay attention to the signals the body sends. When your body needs food, you will get hungry. (It is possible that some of you may *never* have experienced hunger.) Hunger is different from appetite. Appetite is the desire for food, and hunger is the body's need for food. Some examples of hunger are: growling stomach, headache, and loss of concentration. Some examples of appetite are: smelling baked bread, seeing a pie, and reading the menu at a restaurant. You will have to determine how your body "tells" you it's hungry, and then respond to those signals. You should learn to eat only when you are hungry. To be even more precise, you should eat when you are optimally hungry. That sounds strange, doesn't it? It isn't really, but you have to pay attention to the degree of hunger you have. A way to help determine your degree of hunger is to rate it on a scale. For instance, you can use a scale of one to five. A "one" means you are hungry but can wait to eat; a "five" means you are ravenous. If you wait until your hunger is a "five," you may overeat by eating a large amount in a short period of time. On the other hand, if you eat when your hunger is a "one," you probably won't eat enough to satisfy your hunger. Therefore, the most optimal "hunger indicator" is a three or four on the hunger scale. Continue to evaluate your hunger several times throughout the meal. When you are no longer hungry, stop eating!

The second part to this strategy of eating in response to hunger is to eat what will satisfy. You can do this by really tasting your food. That sounds easy enough, and some of you are probably saying, "What are they talking about? Of course, I taste my food." But do you? Try rating the taste of what you eat. Once again the easiest way is to use a scale of one to five. A "one" on the taste scale means you can take it or leave it, and a "five" describes one of the most delicious things you've ever eaten. Why waste the intake of fat and calories on a "one"? You want most of your food to be a "three" or "four" taste. Those foods you will find satisfying, and if you use the hunger scale, you will eat the appropriate amounts. Most of your food choices should be "threes" and "fours," but *don't* deprive yourself of "fives" now and then. We all need some "fives" in our life.

If you use the hunger and taste rating scales, you will begin to take control of your eating and find that you actually start to lose unwanted weight. You may even be surprised to find that foods which are low in cholesterol and saturated fats can also be quite tasty.

Examining other eating habits will give you more ways to obtain and maintain ideal body weight. When? Where? How frequently? How long? These are questions you have to answer about your eating. The answers to these questions may not be as easy as you think, or they may be different from what you think. Let's take a look at these questions one at a time.

When do you eat? Do you always eat at certain times of the day or with a particular activity? For instance, do you have meals at specific times, snack with television watching, or eat at ball games? These are just a few examples of when you eat being determined by factors other than your hunger. When you eat should be in response to your body's need for food and not as a reaction to other circumstances and events.

Where do you eat? If you are eating in front of the TV, at your desk, or in your car, can you be paying attention to what you're eating and how it tastes? You should only eat in places that have been designated appropriate for eating. For instance, the kitchen, the dining room, a cafeteria, or a restaurant are appropriate eating areas. If you limit your eating to those designated places, you will be surprised at how you can decrease your food intake.

How frequently do you eat? Some of you eat virtually every waking hour of the day. (Some of you may even awake during the night to eat.) Once again, if you are eating in response to hunger, you will eliminate this continuous eating pattern. There are two additional considerations involving the frequency of eating. First, do not eat after eight o'clock at night or four hours before going to bed. Remember that food is energy or fuel for the body. When your body is at rest, it uses considerably less energy. Therefore, food that you eat just before going to sleep will not be used, and the body will store it as fat. The second consideration is the importance of eating breakfast. By eating in the morning, your body's metabolism wakes up. The sooner your body starts to work (metabolism increases), the more energy it will use. All of you expert dieters know that if you don't eat breakfast, you can sometimes go until well past noon without feeling hungry. But if you eat breakfast, you start to get hungry about eleven or twelve o'clock. That's because your body's metabolism had to function at a higher rate when you gave it food to digest at breakfast. The fact that you are hungry again means that you have burned up calories, and now the body needs more. So don't skip that nutritious, low-fat breakfast that burns up those calories.

How long do you eat at a meal? Studies have shown that it takes 20-25 minutes for the stomach to send a signal to the brain and for the brain to respond with a signal that you are full. If you eat too quickly, your brain may not get the message it needs, and you will be hungry again very soon. On the other hand, if you take too long to eat, your appetite center in the brain can be restimulated, and you could overeat. Try to keep meals in the 20 minute time frame. If you eat too quickly, you need to prolong your actual eating time. You can do this by putting your silverware down frequently or cutting your food into small pieces and eating them one at a time. Additionally, you can use your napkin between bites or stop eating periodically during the meal. For those of you who eat too slowly, you may need to take smaller portions of food or limit your conversation during a meal.

If you begin to change your incorrect eating habits, you will find that you can lose and/or maintain ideal body weight and make eating more enjoyable. Be patient with yourself. Changing habits takes time. You did not develop your eating behaviors overnight, and you won't be able to change them as quickly as you would wish. When you conquer a bad habit, encourage yourself with a non-food reward such as buying a new book, record, or piece of clothing you've been wanting; indulging in an extra long bath or walk; or taking time to enjoy some special thing or activity. It's important to reward yourself for an accomplishment!

LIMITING CHOLESTEROL WILL HELP CONTROL BLOOD LIPIDS

As you have read in previous chapters, limiting your intake of cholesterol will help control your blood lipids. Remember that cholesterol is found in foods from animal sources. Additionally, high concentrations of cholesterol are contained in the organ meat of animals and in the skin of fowl. Therefore, it is very important that your intake of these foods be limited. The recommendation from the American Heart Association is that cholesterol intake be limited to no more than 250-300 mg. of cholesterol per day. This is known as the AHA Step 1 diet for cholesterol control. If a person is restricting cholesterol to 250–300 mg. a day and limiting fat intake to 30% of his calories, and still has not obtained a total blood cholesterol level of 200 mg./dL, further action must be taken. Limiting the cholesterol intake to 250–300 mg. a day may not be enough of a limitation in some individuals to successfully lower their blood cholesterol. The American Heart Association has dietary restrictions that are referred to as Step

II diet control for those who do not reach acceptable blood cholesterol levels with the Step I diet. The Step II diet limits cholesterol intake to 150-200 mg. a day and further decreases saturated fat in the diet. These diets will be discussed in more detail later in this chapter. It is important to remember that limiting cholesterol intake is only one step in the process of lowering blood lipids. Other measures include lowering the amount of saturated fats in your diet and increasing the unsaturated fats that you eat. These steps, in combination with maintaining ideal body weight, regular exercise, stopping smoking, and adhering to any medication program your physician may prescribe, will give you the best defense in fighting cholesterol.

REGULAR PHYSICAL ACTIVITY

Exercise is another part of the total plan to improve your cholesterol status. Studies have shown that regular physical exercise increases the amount of HDL cholesterol and lowers LDL cholesterol. The key to a successful exercise program is that it must be something you can and will do forever. That means it has to be enjoyable for you. If you hate to walk, don't start a walking program. There are several activities that are beneficial to the cardiovascular system and will increase the HDL cholesterol. Choose the activity that is best suited to you and your lifestyle. If you have not been physically active, you should consult your physician before starting any program. Exercise should be done at least three times a week for fifteen to twenty minutes. The excuse that you just don't have time for a regular exercise program is a poor one. Isn't your life and health worth 45 to 60 minutes a week? Start slowly and build up your endurance. You will not be able to exercise for 15-20 minutes continuously the first time. The point is not to overexercise but to develop a routine of regular physical activity.

Some of the exercises that are good for your cardiovascular health are: walking, jogging, bicycling, swimming, jumping rope, and dancing. Remember that whatever activity you choose, it should be one that you will be able to do for 15–20 minutes at a time. If you have knee problems or live in an area that you cannot get out and walk, then perhaps a stationary bike would be best for you. If you don't have access to a pool, don't choose swimming as your activity. The most important part of any physical activity program is that you do it consistently. Start today and stay with it for life.

STOP SMOKING *NOW!!!*

Smoking is one of the major contributors to cardiovascular disease and heart attack (in addition to its cancer causing effects). The effects of smoking are cumulative. That means if you have never smoked, you are better off than someone who smoked for five years and has stopped. If you smoked for ten years, you have had more damage than someone who smoked for five, but less than someone who smoked for twenty. To be even more practical, if you quit smoking today, you will have less damage than if you quit tomorrow. Smoking does have an effect on the body's cholesterol and triglyceride levels. Smokers have lower HDL cholesterol and more LDL cholesterol. If you want to do everything you can to improve your cholesterol level and decrease your risk of heart attack, you will stop smoking in addition to following the diet recommended in this book.

Stopping smoking isn't easy, *but it can be done! There are more than 35 million Americans who are ex-smokers. If they could all succeed, so can you. About 70% of all ex-*

smokers had failed at least once before successfully quitting, so don't use the old excuse that you've tried. People either quit abruptly or gradually cut back. Statistics show 90% of all people who have successfully quit have done so "cold turkey". But to do this, you may need some strategies to help you along. Try to determine *why* you smoke. Do you like the taste? If so, find and substitute something that is just as satisfying for you (and low-fat). Try mints, gum, or hard candy. Do you like the relaxing feeling smoking gives you? Substitute deep breathing and imagery instead of a cigarette. Are you the kind of individual who uses a cigarette to keep your hands occupied? Replace that cigarette with a paperclip, rubber band, pencil, or marbles (like Captain Queeg). Go to movies, museums, department stores, or any place that prohibits smoking while you are trying to quit. Finally, watch what non-smokers and ex-smokers are doing and imitate them when you feel the need for a cigarette. Talk to ex-smokers to find out what helped them. Put down those cigarettes right now and help raise your HDL cholesterol level and your overall health!

FOLLOW YOUR DOCTOR'S ADVICE

The best and first treatment choice for lowering cholesterol is always diet. But sometimes diet alone can't sufficiently reduce the cholesterol. In those cases, drug therapy will be added. Medications are never a substitute for diet. As a matter of fact, a diet that is high in saturated fats and cholesterol can minimize the beneficial effects of the drug therapy. When your physician prescribes a cholesterol lowering medication, it is out of necessity. Medications in combination with the low-fat, low cholesterol diet recommendations are yet another way to help win the war with cholesterol. (We will be covering the various lipid lowering medications in the next chapter.)

To help control cholesterol, you should obtain and maintain ideal body weight, stop smoking, establish and adhere to a regular exercise program, and take any lipid lowering medications that have been prescribed by your physician. All of these steps need to be done in addition to following the low saturated fat, low cholesterol diet that the AHA recommends. Following all of these suggestions will help you do all that you can to control your cholesterol. Cholesterol is a killer, so take all of the steps you can to conquer it.

9 When Diet Alone Isn't Enough

In some people, following the recommendations of a low saturated fat and low cholesterol diet may not be enough to sufficiently reduce their cholesterol to an acceptable range. Those individuals may require prescription lipid lowering medications. When medication is required, it is *always in addition to dietary control.* It has been shown that the beneficial effect of the medications can be reduced if a person continues to eat a diet high in saturated fats. For this reason, it is important to continue with the kind of dietary changes that are found in this book and coincide with the recommendations of the AHA.

If medication is necessary, what kind of drug therapy is prescribed? Generally, the first step a physician will take is to use a type of medication called a bile acid sequestrant. There are two medications in this category. They are Questran and Colestid. These agents work in the intestinal tract and are not absorbed by the body. Questran and Colestid trap cholesterol in the intestine like a sponge soaking up water. They "hold" the cholesterol and eliminate it from the body in the stool. These medications lower total cholesterol and LDL, but they do not reduce

73

triglyceride levels. Bile acid sequestrants generally lower total cholesterol by about 9% and LDL cholesterol by nearly 12%. In the Lipid Research Clinics Coronary Primary Prevention Trial (LRC CPPT), Questran was the medication used in those men who did not receive a placebo. The LRC CPPT showed that the 9% reduction in the total cholesterol resulted in a 19% reduction in the incidence of coronary heart disease.

Are there side effects for this type of medication? The bile acid sequestrants are safe medications; however, they do have some side effects that people find uncomfortable and/or unpleasant. Because Questran and Colestid work in the intestinal tract and are excreted in the stool, the most common side effects are associated with gastrointestinal discomfort. Bloating, indigestion, gas, and constipation are the most common side effects. These side effects occur because bile, which contains the cholesterol in the intestine, is trapped by the medications and eliminated in the stool. Bile is a digestive aid and serves as an irritant to the bowel. Adding fruits, vegetables, and high fiber grains to the diet will help reduce or eliminate these gastrointestinal side effects.

In addition to the gastrointestinal side effects, Questran and Colestid trap and eliminate some medications that you may be taking. Therefore, Questran and Colestid should *not* be taken on the same time schedule as other medications. It is generally recommended that other medications be taken at least one hour before, or four to six hours after taking the Questran and/or Colestid. Ask your doctor about how to most effectively take all of your medications. As with all medicines these should not be stopped abruptly without your physician's knowledge and permission.

What if the bile acid sequestrant medications don't work? Is there anything else that could be prescribed?

Nicotinic acid can be added to the regimen of diet and Questran or Colestid. Nicotinic acid is a B vitamin. In doses that are far larger than those needed as a vitamin, nicotinic acid lowers LDL and it's precursor, VLDL (very low density lipoprotein). Nicotinic acid decreases the production of VLDL in the body. Since LDL is made from VLDL, the LDL level is lowered when production of VLDL is decreased. Nicotinic acid can effectively lower cholesterol levels; however, to achieve those effects requires taking 3 to 4 1/2 grams every day. Nicotinic acid is available in 100 and 500 mg. tablets. This means that it would be necessary to take between 6 and 45 tablets per day depending on the tablet and dose prescribed.

What are the side effects of nicotinic acid? Flushing is the most common side effect. Generalized itching and gastric irritation do occur as side effects in some people as well. This medication is an acid, and people who have ulcers or any gastrointestinal irritation and bleeding should inform their physician before starting on nicotinic acid. To reduce the side effects, the dose is started at a low level and gradually increased. In addition to dose regulation, taking an aspirin about 30 minutes before the nicotinic acid reduces the flushing and itching that occur. Large doses of nicotinic acid can also cause problems with liver function and even lead to liver failure. In addition, nicotinic acid can cause irregular heart rhythm. Even though nicotinic acid is a non-prescription medication, it should only be used under the supervision of a physician.

What are second line medications and when would they be prescribed? Lorelco and Lopid are both considered to be second step lipid lowering medications. Lorelco could be used in a person who did not achieve an acceptable reduction in cholesterol with the use of diet and a bile acid sequestrant with or without nicotinic acid. The second line medications can also be used in someone who could not tolerate the first line medications. Lorelco lowers LDL cholesterol but does not have an effect on the triglycerides. The therapeutic results from the use of Lorelco are variable. Some people have an excellent result with a 25% reduction in their LDL cholesterol, while others can achieve only a 5% lowering of LDL. Lorelco lowers the HDL as well as the LDL cholesterol and, therefore, should be used cautiously. The side effects of Lorelco are primarily gastrointestinal, and include diarrhea, nausea, and gas.

Lopid is a medication that primarily lowers triglyceride levels. The total cholesterol and LDL are mildly reduced, but Lopid does cause a significant increase in the HDL cholesterol. Lopid is not currently approved by the FDA for use in lowering serum cholesterol, but that may soon change because of the results of a recent cholesterol study. The Helsinki Study involved 4,081 men in a study comparing a placebo to Lopid. The results showed that total cholesterol was reduced 8%, and LDL cholesterol was also reduced by 8%. Triglycerides were reduced by 35%, and HDL cholesterol *increased* by 10%. The end result was that the group of men taking the Lopid had a 34% reduction in coronary heart disease when compared to the men taking the placebo. As with any individual study, one should be careful to not jump to unsubstantiated conclusions. However, it appears that raising HDL cholesterol, in addition to lowering LDL cholesterol and triglycerides, is beneficial. Future studies will provide more information about this medication.

Lopid does not have many side effects. Most people can tolerate this medication without difficulty. The incidence of nausea and diarrhea, which are the primary side effects, are low. Lopid is not currently considered a first line medication in the treatment of elevated cholesterol.

THE NEWEST MEDICATION IN THE FIGHT AGAINST CHOLESTEROL

The newest medication available to help lower cholesterol levels is lovastatin. It is unlike any of the cholesterol controlling medications that we have previously discussed. In Chapter 1, you learned that the body can make cholesterol, which is necessary for certain essential bodily functions. The primary production site for this endogeneous cholesterol is the liver. The liver makes about 70% of all the cholesterol produced by the body. This production of cholesterol is how your body guarantees that it will always have enough cholesterol. Lovastatin blocks the production of cholesterol in the liver by stopping the action of a necessary enzyme. When the liver is prohibited from making cholesterol, absorption of cholesterol from the blood is increased to meet the body's demands. The liver increases its absorption of cholesterol from the blood by increasing the number of places that LDL can be received into the liver. Since the liver is removing LDL cholesterol from the blood, there is less LDL cholesterol left in the blood. In studies, lovastatin reduces serum LDL cholesterol by about 40%, and total cholesterol by 30–35%. There has also been an associated increase in the HDL cholesterol in people taking lovastatin, but it is a minimal increase of only 5–9%. Lovastatin does a remarkable job of lowering LDL and total cholesterol. Unlike some of the other cholesterol lowering medications, it does not seem to interfere with other medications taken at the same time.

Lovastatin is an exciting new type of medication that can be used to help control cholesterol. However, there are some precautions that must be considered. With the development of a medication which can lower LDL cholesterol by almost 50%, many people think that they can "just take a pill" and cure their cholesterol problems. This simply isn't true. This medication, like all of the others we have discussed, must be used in combination with a low saturated fat, low cholesterol diet to be effective. Since cholesterol control must be for a lifetime, it is very important to follow a low cholesterol, low saturated fat diet rather than depend on a medication alone. Lovastatin, like the majority of the cholesterol lowering medications, is expensive. Its long term use can have a significant financial burden on the user. This is another reason to try to control cholesterol with diet alone or with diet and minimal amounts of medication.

Lovastatin does seem to have a bright future, but we must state that, to date, it has not been used as widely or studied as extensively as other medications used for cholesterol control. The long-term history of the drug and information that is accumulated from its use by many thousands of people is not currently available. All medications have side effects as well as beneficial effects, and lovastatin is no exception. The two side effects that have received the most attention are an increase in the liver enzymes and increased opacity of the lens of the eye. Exactly what these side effects will lead to long term, no one can say at this time. The increased liver enzymes, which occur in about 1% of people, may mean that the liver is working too hard and could possibly fail as a result of this overwork. For this reason, blood tests to check liver function are recommended at regular intervals when the medication is first started. If elevations are found, the lovastatin is stopped and usually causes no harm. The increased opacity of the lens of the eye may make the person susceptible to cataracts. Studies are currently in progress to determine if these lens opacifications have any significance. To date, no effect on vision has ever been reported because of the use of lovastatin.

In review, lovastatin is the most recent medication available for the control of cholesterol. It has the potential to reduce LDL cholesterol by 40–50%. This medication, in addition to diet control, could significantly lower a person's cholesterol into a safe range. While lovastatin appears to be an effective medication with few side effects, it is a relatively new medication that will require large-scale, long-term studies to adequately test its safety.

The last part of this chapter is optional reading. The information that follows represents the current recommendation of an expert panel of the National Cholesterol Education Program. This information represents the guidelines for treatment that were sent to all physicians. These guidelines have been simplified in this chapter to make them more understandable. They are presented so that you know what the experts have recommended concerning detection and treatment of hyperlipidemia.

PROFILE OF CURRENTLY USED
LIPID-LOWERING AGENTS

Drugs	Total Cholesterol	LDL Cholesterol	HDL Cholesterol	Triglycerides
Gemfibrozil Capsules, USP (Lopid®)	↓	↓	↑ ↑	↓ ↓
Lovastatin (Mevacor®)	↓ ↓	↓ ↓	↔	↓
Cholestyramine Resin Powder (Questran®)	↓ ↓	↓ ↓	↔	↑
Colestipol HCl Granules (Colestid®)	↓ ↓	↓ ↓	↔	↑
Probucol Tablets (Lorelco®)	↓ ↓	↓ ↓	↓	↔
Niacin Tablets (nicotinic acid) (Nicolar®)	↓	↓	↑ or ↓	↓ ↓

LDL, low-density lipoprotein; HDL, high-density lipoprotein; VLDL, very-low-density lipoprotein
↑, increase; ↑↑, greater increase; ↓, decrease; ↓↓, greater decrease; ↔, no effect

EFFECT OF MEDICATION ON SPECIFIC BLOOD LIPIDS

DRUG	PRIMARY EFFECTS ON PLASMA LIPIDS AND LIPOPROTEINS	PRINCIPAL ADVERSE REACTIONS AND DRUG INTERACTIONS
Gemfibrozil Capsules, USP (Lopid®)	Triglycerides ↓↓ Cholesterol ↓ VLDL ↓↓ LDL ↓ HDL ↑↑	Abdominal and epigastric pain, diarrhea, nausea, vomiting Known interaction with anticoagulants
Cholestyramine Resin Powder (Questran®)	Triglycerides ↑ Cholesterol ↓↓ VLDL ↑ LDL ↓↓ HDL ↔	Constipation, nausea, bloating Decreased absorption of fat-soluable vitamins (A, D, and K) and other drugs, delaying or reducing their absorption
Colestipol HCl Granules (Colestid®)	Triglycerides ↑ Cholesterol ↓↓ VLDL ↑ LDL ↓↓ HDL ↔	Constipation, nausea, bloating Decreased absorption of fat-soluable vitamins (A, D, and K) and other drugs, delaying or reducing their absorption
Probucol Tablets (Lorelco®)	Triglycerides ↔ Cholesterol ↓↓ VLDL ↔ LDL ↓↓ HDL ↓	Diarrhea, abdominal pain, nausea Headache, rash Prolongation of QT interval Decreases HDL cholesterol
Niacin Tablets (nicotinic acid) (Nicolar®)	Triglycerides ↓↓ Cholesterol ↓ VLDL ↓↓ LDL ↓ HDL ↑ or ↓	Severe, generalized flushing Pruritus/dry skin GI disorders Hyperuricemia Abnormal liver function tests
Lovastatin (Mevacor®)	Triglycerides ↓ Cholesterol ↓↓ VLDL ↓ LDL ↓↓ HDL ↔	Nausea, gas, diarrhea, constipation, abdominal pain, dyspepsia, rash, headache Lens opacities—slit lamp tests recommended at start of treatment and once a year thereafter Liver function tests recommended every 4–6 weeks for at least 15 months of treatment

Apo, apolipoprotein; HDL, high-density lipoprotein; LDL, low-density lipoprotein; VLDL, very-low-density lipoprotein; ↑, increase; ↑↑, greater increase; ↓, decrease; ↓↓, greater decrease; ↔, no effect

CURRENT RECOMMENDATIONS

The 1987 report of the National Cholesterol Education Program Expert Panel on Detection, Evaluation, and Treatment of High Blood Cholesterol in Adults made specific recommendations to all physicians concerning evaluation and treatment of blood cholesterol levels. These recommendations are presented here in verbal form and in Appendix 3 in flow chart form. Reading the written explanation and then referring to the flow chart will make understanding the recommendations easier. In addition, the flow chart will be easier to refer to for future reference once the information below is read and understood. These guidelines, from this panel of national experts, were sent to all physicians in the United States.

Initial Classification

- Every adult age 20 and over should have a nonfasting total blood cholesterol level.
- All blood cholesterol levels above 200 mg./dL should be repeated, and the average used to guide clinical decisions.
- Coronary Heart Disease (CHD) risk factors as defined in this report include:
  - Male sex
  - Family history of heart attack or sudden death before age 55 in a parent or brother or sister
  - Cigarette smoking (currently smoke more than 10 cigarettes per day)
  - High blood pressure
  - Low HDL Cholesterol (below 35 mg./dL on two different measurements)

- Diabetes
- History of stroke or peripheral vascular disease (blockages in leg arteries)
- Severe obesity (greater than 30% overweight) (see ideal body weight chart)
- All patients with a level of 240 mg./dL or higher should have a fasting lipid profile performed.
- Patients with a level of 200-239 mg./dL and definite CHD or two CHD risk factors should have a fasting lipid profile performed.
- Patients with a level of 200-239 mg./dL and no CHD and one or less CHD risk factors should be provided with Step 1 AHA diet and have cholesterol checked at least once a year.
- Patients with a level of greater than 200 mg./dL should be provided general dietary information and risk factor education. Cholesterol should be rechecked within 5 years.

Classification Based on LDL Cholesterol

If a fasting lipid profile was recommended above, dietary or drug therapy is decided on the LDL cholesterol levels. A fasting specimen should be at least a 12-hour fast with total cholesterol, HDL cholesterol, and triglycerides measured. An average of 2 to 3 measurements over 1 to 8 weeks should be made for decision-making purposes.

- If LDL level is less than 130 mg./dL, general dietary and risk factor education should be given and total cholesterol remeasured within 5 years.

- If LDL level is 130–159 mg./dL and no CHD and one or less CHD risk factors, then Step 1 AHA diet and recheck total cholesterol annually.

- If LDL level is greater than or equal to 160 mg./dL or 130–159 with CHD or two CHD risk factors, patient should have clinical evaluation and LDL goal set. LDL goal is less than 160 mg./dL or less than 130 mg./dL if CHD or two CHD risk factors are present.

Dietary Treatment

If the LDL cholesterol is above the recommended guidelines, then the first step is always dietary therapy.

- Instruct on Step 1 AHA diet and remeasure total cholesterol in 4 to 6 weeks and at 3 months. The recommendation is for the total cholesterol to be less than 240 mg./dL or less than 200 mg./dL if CHD or two CHD risk factors are present. If the total cholesterol goal is met, then the LDL cholesterol should be checked to confirm reaching the LDL goal. If the LDL goal is met, then the cholesterol should be remeasured 4 times in the first year and twice a year thereafter. Dietary and behavior modifications should be reinforced.

- If the cholesterol goal is not met, then the patient should be referred to a registered dietician for counselling and retrial on Step 1 diet. If cholesterol goal is still not met, then Step 2 diet should be used. A minimum of 6 months of diet is used to obtain cholesterol goals. Cholesterol levels should be checked every 6 to 12 weeks while trying to obtain the goals. If cholesterol goal is met, LDL level should be determined to see if LDL goal is met. If LDL goal is met, do long term monitoring as noted at the end of the previous paragraph.

- If the cholesterol goal is not achieved, consider drug therapy.

Drug Therapy

- Maximal efforts at dietary therapy should be made before initiating drug therapy and should be continued even if drug therapy is needed.
- The panel set the LDL levels at which drug treatment is started in such a way as to create a protective barrier to the inappropriate overuse of cholesterol-lowering drugs.
- Patients with LDL cholesterol of 190 mg./dL or greater, and those with LDL cholesterol 160—189 mg./dL who also have CHD or two CHD risk factors, should be considered for drug therapy.
- The bile acid sequestrants and nicotinic acid are considered the drugs of first choice. Both Questran and nicotinic acid have been shown to lower CHD risk in clinical trials, and their long term safety has been established.
- Lovastatin is the first of a new class of drugs. These drugs are very effective in lowering LDL cholesterol, but their effect on CHD incidence and their long-term safety have yet to be established.
- The other available drugs—Lorelco, Lopid, and Colestid—are not as effective in lowering LDL cholesterol as are the drugs of first choice or lovastatin.
- The goals of drug therapy are the same as those of dietary therapy.
- Drug therapy is likely to continue for a lifetime.
- Cholesterol is an active area of research. Ongoing and future investigations can be expected to expand and refine drug treatment options.

- If cholesterol goal is not achieved with diet and a first line drug, then a different drug or combination should be used. If cholesterol goal is still not reached, a lipid specialist should be consulted.

- If LDL goal is achieved on drug therapy, then total cholesterol should be monitored every 4 months and LDL measured annually.

- Each person is different, so treatment, both diets and medicines, should be individualized. Overall coronary heart disease risk status should be carefully monitored and changed where appropriate.

10 Eating Away From Home

Eating away from home is a common part of the American lifestyle. This may be due to established routines, necessity, convenience, or for pleasure. Whatever the reason, you can certainly continue eating out and maintain the healthy low-fat diet you've worked to establish. In many ways eating a low-fat meal away from home has become easier in recent years. With the increased awareness of cholesterol and saturated fats, many patrons of restaurants have been requesting low-fat food selections. Today, you will find in many restaurants and on some airlines, meals that follow the American Heart Association guidelines. These approved items or meals have some special designation on the menu. When you see these items, usually designated by an "AHA approved" or a heart on the menu, it will be easy for you to select a low-fat meal away from home. But what if the restaurant of your choice doesn't have these menu keys? Don't despair. With a little thought and planning, you can make selections which follow the guidelines you have learned in this book.

Here are a few suggestions to remember when you go to a restaurant for a low-fat meal. Everything you have learned to this point still applies. You may want to phone the restaurant before going, to inquire if they have low-fat, low cholesterol menu items or if they are willing to substitute on request. Once you arrive, take your time to examine the menu. Choose items that contain polyunsaturates and are low in saturated fats. As a patron of the restaurant, you are the customer, and the customer is *Always* right. Don't be intimidated by the menu, the surroundings, or the personnel. Ask how food is prepared and request any necessary changes. If you have made a particular request and the food is not prepared or served accordingly, you should send it back. Be assertive, not aggressive, in your requests. This chapter will provide you with guidelines on how to eat away from home while continuing to adhere to a good low saturated fat diet.

If the restaurant does not have healthy-heart food choices, you should request that they consider adding these types of meals to their menus.

WHAT TO LOOK FOR ON THE MENU

There are certain words or phrases that are used to describe food preparation that will help you spot low-fat selections. The following lists are quick references. The first two lists include descriptions and methods of food preparation which should be low in saturated fat. The last two lists describe some methods of food preparation which are most likely to be poor low-fat food choices. The remainder of this chapter will give you more detailed information on restaurant eating. Included will be information on all types of dining, from fast food to elegant restaurants and ethnic eateries.

CHOOSE THESE METHODS OF FOOD PREPARATION

Baked
Broiled
Poached
Roasted
Steamed

SELECT THESE DESCRIPTIONS OF PREPARATION

In Wine
Tomato Juice
Dry broiled (in lemon juice or wine)
Fresh from the garden

AVOID SELECTIONS WITH THE FOLLOWING
DESCRIPTIONS

Fried, Pan fried, or in its own Gravy
Braised
Buttered, Buttery, or in Butter Sauce
Creamy, Creamed, in Cream Sauce, or Hollandaise
Crispy
Cheese Sauce, Escalloped, Au Gratin, Parmesan,
    or Cheesy
Basted, Sautéed or Marinated in Oil or Butter

TYPES OF DISHES TO AVOID

Casseroles
Hash
Meat or Pot Pies
Stews

HOW TO BEGIN TO CHOOSE

Sometimes, with all of the many choices presented on
a menu, it is rather easy to be a bit overwhelmed and

confused. Don't panic or worry. The exact same rules for a good low saturated fat diet that you have been learning all along still apply. If you will be selecting several courses, it is probably wise to make your entree choice first. Even though you may be having an appetizer, salad, or soup first, don't make that your first selection from the menu. You will find it easier to select the entree and build the rest of the meal around it. That means that you will want to choose an entree that is preferably turkey, chicken, fish, or non-meat. You will find it best to limit your perusal of the menu to just those items. Looking at menu items that you have no intention of selecting tends to make the decision process more difficult than it needs to be. Examine the entree items that fit the low-fat category and determine how they are prepared. Continue to think about saturated fats just as you do when grocery shopping. The part of the menu that describes the preparation is like looking at the ingredient list on a label. (And we all know that you're now a pro at label reading!) If the menu does not describe the preparation process, ask your server. Remember, you are the customer! If the item is prepared in a way that makes it an unwise low-fat choice, you may be able to request a change in preparation. Low-fat eating is becoming more of a norm in the United States, and restaurants are frequently asked to alter the preparation of menu items, so don't be bashful. You are not the first and won't be the last patron to make that request. An example of preparation substitution might be a breast of chicken that is broiled with wine and butter. Certainly, the breast of chicken is a low saturated fat choice, and broiled with wine would be an excellent selection. The butter in addition to the wine adds unnecessary saturated fats to this item. Ask the server if the same selection could be prepared without the butter, using just wine or replacing the butter with margarine. If those changes in preparation can be accommodated, then the item would be a wise choice.

If you select an entree that is simple in its preparation it is probably a better low-fat choice. Choose items that are broiled or baked and have a simple but tasty basting. Healthful, low-fat meals can be tasty and delicious, so don't settle for anything less. Pick your entree first and remember to limit menu gazing to just the selections that are good low-fat choices. Now that the entree has been chosen, go back and select the rest of the meal.

Choosing the Rest of the Meal

After the entree has been selected, it is easier for most people to choose the rest of the meal. Salads are excellent low-fat, low calorie additions, or sometimes a meal in themselves. Greens, vegetables, and fruits make delicious, low-fat salads. Stay away from eggs, meats, and toppings like bacon and croutons. The popularity of salad bars has made it possible for you to be selective in the creation of your salad, and many offer a wide variety of choices. If a salad bar is not available, you may request that eggs, meat, bacon or croutons be eliminated in the preparation, or simply remove the unwanted items from your salad when it arrives. When ordering a salad, request that the dressing be served on the side. You will then be able to control the amount that is added. Often a perfectly good and healthful salad is drowned in a high calorie, high fat dressing. Try lemon juice or oil and vinegar as dressings. When using a rich dressing, add a little lemon juice, vinegar, or water to dilute it and use sparingly. Salads can be an excellent low-fat, low cholesterol accompaniment to any meal. Enjoy!

Do Appetizers Fit into a Healthful Low-Fat Meal?

Absolutely! You can enjoy fresh fruits and melons or raw vegetables as appetizers. Additionally, steamed or raw seafood is an excellent choice for starting a meal. There is no need to deprive yourself of an appetizer if you are on a low-fat food plan. Just pick the ones that are appropriate. A word of caution to those of you who must watch your calorie intake to achieve or maintain your ideal weight. You may want to think twice about using calories on an appetizer and "save" them for the main event, or even dessert. The choice is yours, so decide which will give you the most satisfaction. If you do decide to start your meal with an appetizer, vegetables may satisfy your need without spending too much of your calorie allowance.

Appetizers can make an evening of dining out an even more special event. There are many low-fat choices that you can enjoy and continue to eat for a healthy heart. You will want to stay away from crackers, spreads, and chips. As you have seen in some of the label reading, these items tend to contain hydrogenated fats and often palm and/or coconut oil. Choose your appetizers wisely for both fat and calorie content, and get ready to have a wonderful time. Enjoy your meal!

Soup as Part of a Low-Fat Diet

There are many wonderful soups you can enjoy, but you must be careful. You can prepare almost any soup at home by substituting ingredients and altering the preparation, but soup selections can be a bit tricky when eating out. (See the recipes contained in Chapter 11 for additional information.) There are some problems that you should consider when ordering a soup in a restaurant. First of all, you can not make requests for the soup to be prepared in a specific way, as you often can with other parts of the meal. The reason for this is that soups are made in a large quantity and are served in portions from the pot. This means that you will not be able to have your soup prepared with skim milk instead of whole milk or heavy cream. Therefore, soups that are listed as "creamed", "cream of", or "creamy" should be avoided when making your selection. Soups frequently contain ingredients that are prepared with fats and/or egg yolks. For example, soups containing noodles, dumplings, or matzo balls probably contain fats and eggs and should not be selected when dining out. Soup selection in a restaurant can be done; it just requires a little discrimination and thought. If you have any questions about the preparation of the soup, ask your server. The information you receive will help you make a better choice.

There are many soups that are good, low-fat choices in restaurants and many, many more that you can make at home. Once again, limit your consideration of the menu to only the soups that would be wise low-fat, low cholesterol choices. You can select from either hot or cold soups. Hot soup on a cold day can be something that is especially good and satisfying. And cold soups can really hit the spot in the heat of the summer. Choose a soup that is clear or is listed as a broth or a consommé on the menu. These are usually good low-fat soups. Most of the cold fruit and vegetable soups are good low-fat choices as long as they are not creamed. Soup selections when dining out are more limited than with home preparation, but you can certainly have a good satisfying bowl of soup with your meal.

Bread and Butter

Perhaps the old adage "bread and butter" referring to something pure and simple will be changing. Neither bread, and certainly not butter, is pure when you are thinking cholesterol. You already know that butter has both cholesterol and saturated fat and should be avoided. But what about bread? When eating out, limit your use of breads. Most breads do contain eggs, milk, and butter. Once again, you will have many more options when baking at home. For example, you can replace whole eggs with egg whites or egg substitutes, skim milk can be used instead of whole milk, and margarine can be used in place of butter in your recipes. (See recipes in Chapter 11 for further information.) When eating at a restaurant, you do not have to give up the bread or breadsticks, but use your judgement and limit how much you eat. If you do eat the bread, avoid using butter. Ask for margarine and use it sparingly. Both the bread and margarine contain calories that you may prefer eating in the entree, dessert, or beverage. The choice is yours to make, so "spend" your calories in the way that will give you the most pleasure. Bread, breadsticks, and margarine can all be enjoyed when dining at home or out, but eat them in moderation.

Rolls, pastry, and Danish all belong to the "bread" family but are generally worse for you than bread. These items generally contain more butter and sometimes additional egg yolks. Additionally, some rolls, pastry, and Danish contain cheese. Obviously, all of these items should be avoided or at least limited.

Would You Care for a Dessert?

Sure, why not! You can have a wonderful low cholesterol, low-fat dessert without feeling deprived or self-sacrificing. With the increased awareness of cholesterol, you will find that dessert items on the menu have changed in recent years. How many times have you ended a perfectly delicious meal by over-indulging in a high-fat dessert? Do you remember how you felt after eating that dessert? All too often, desserts with lots of whipped cream, chocolate, or sauces make you uncomfortable. When that happens, you find that you didn't really enjoy the dessert after all. You can eliminate that too-full feeling by choosing a low-fat, low cholesterol dessert to top off your meal to perfection. You don't have to eliminate dessert as there are plenty of good low-fat choices available. One way you can enjoy dessert is by finishing your meal with fresh fruit. Please don't add whipped cream or toppings, either dairy or nondairy. Many of the dairy toppings are made from whole milk and cream. The nondairy toppings frequently contain palm or coconut oils. Fresh fruit finishes your meal with a nice sweet taste without adding fats or a lot of calories. Choosing an out-of-season fruit or an exotic variety may be just the special touch that your dining out experience should have.

You don't want fruit for dessert? There are other good low-fat choices for you. Maybe a cool refreshing ice or sherbet will suit your taste. Or how about an angel food cake with or without fruit topping? These are all good low cholesterol, low-fat desserts you can enjoy. Remember that your selection for desserts prepared at home are increased one hundred fold by making appropriate substitutions and preparations in the recipe. But eating out can still offer you good dessert selection. Go ahead, order dessert, and sit back and relax after that wonderful healthy-heart meal you've just enjoyed.

What About Drinks?

Many times drinks are not mentioned when discussing cholesterol. However, there are some cholesterol considerations. The first consideration is that alcoholic beverages add calories. Alcohol does not contain cholesterol or saturated fat, but it does contain calories. You know that one important way to lower and control cholesterol is by maintaining ideal body weight. You may certainly choose to have an alcoholic beverage, but you must adjust your meal to accommodate the additional calories. You may want to minimize the calories by diluting the alcohol; that way you can enjoy more for less. One way to do just that is by drinking a wine spritzer instead of a glass of wine. When the wine is diluted with a low calorie seltzer or soda, you can reduce the calorie content to almost one half and still have all of the enjoyment. If you do not want to use your calories on alcohol but you want to have something that is fun and delicious, you may try a low calorie sparkling water with a lime, lemon, or orange slice.

In addition to the calorie aspect of the alcoholic beverage, you must remember that alcohol raises triglyceride levels. If you have elevated triglycerides, you should avoid alcohol or at least dilute it as we have suggested above. You can dilute wine and "hard liquor," but most people do not dilute beer. Light beers still raise the triglyceride level in your blood. Only the calories are reduced. It is the reduction of calories that allows the beer to be labeled as light. You will have to read the label to determine the calorie content, as each product is a bit different. The fact that alcohol raises triglycerides must be considered when discussing a low cholesterol, low-fat diet.

The final consideration when ordering an alcoholic beverage is to avoid the popular ice cream drinks and specialty liquors. While the piña colada may taste good, it is not good for your heart. Not only is it made with ice cream, but it also contains coconut, both of which are high in saturated fat. Remember that ice cream contains saturated fat whether it is in a bowl or in a drink. To follow a healthful low-fat diet plan you should avoid ice cream drinks because they are sources of saturated fat, as well as cholesterol. Specialty liquors such as Irish cream may in fact contain cream or milk products. You should check the labels of your favorite liquors and find substitutions if they contain these cholesterol raising ingredients. A no-fat spritzer or soda can be the perfect accompaniment to any meal at home or while dining out.

Fast Food Restaurants

It is confusing, and in some cases almost impossible, to try to figure out how much fat is in a fast food item and how it is prepared. We have included an extensive listing of fast food restaurants in the appendix. Restaurants are listed with their menu items and the fat content for the items. You will find it helpful and easy to look up any particular item for a food chain by referring to the tables in Appendix 5. But here are some general tips to remember about fast food eating and the selections you will make.

If you are going to be eating out at a fast food restaurant, there's no need to complain that the menu contains no items low in fat and cholesterol. Most of the national fast food restaurant chains have selections that can fit into a low cholesterol, low-fat diet. Changing times have given you alternatives to the "greasy" fast foods we used to associate with these places. Most fast food establishments now have salads offered on their menus, either prepared or as salad bars. Take advantage of the salad bars to create your own low-fat salad or meal. Remember to stay away from the eggs, meats, bacon, and croutons. At a salad bar you can add the exact amount of dressing you want. Once again, oil and vinegar or lemon juice are the best low-fat dressings. There are some restaurants that offer low-fat and/or low calorie dressings, and these may be good choices for you. Even when the salad is prepared and served to you, the dressing is usually contained in a packet and served on the side. Many of these packets list the ingredients so you can analyze the contents for yourself.

Salads aren't the only new item on fast food menus. You can now get vegetables and baked potatoes instead of the old standard french fries. If you do choose the baked potato, top it with margarine or yogurt in place of the butter and sour cream. Some fast food restaurants also offer baked potatoes topped with vegetables. The vegetables are great as long as they don't come with cheese sauce.

There have been many chicken products added to the fast food menu. But not all of these additions are as healthful as the advertisers would have you think. Chicken products served at fast food eateries are sometimes fried in beef fat and lard. (Check the tables in the appendix.) If that is the case, stay away from the chicken at these places. Chicken that is fried in vegetable oil is better than that fried in beef fat or lard, but not by much. The chicken is still fried, and you know that is not a good low-fat method of preparation. Baked breast of chicken sandwiches are found at some fast food restaurants, and these would be the best choice if available.

When eating at fast food restaurants, stay away from the hamburgers, especially those that are fried. Cheeseburgers are a poor choice because they add more saturated fat in the cheese, in addition to the beef, which may be fried. You can request skim milk at most fast food places if you want a milk product. The milk shakes and malts are to be avoided.

Fast food eating is improving. It is much easier to eat a low-fat meal today at a fast food restaurant than it was even two or three years ago. As the general public becomes more aware of cholesterol, you will probably see additional changes in the menus at fast food places. Speak up and let the big companies know you want to be able to get a fast low-fat meal at their restaurants. Changes have been made because of public demand, and certainly, still more will be made. Remember, you are the customer!

Italian Food

If you think pasta when you say Italian, you are thinking low-fat, low cholesterol foods. Pastas can be good items for the cholesterol conscious eater as long as the pasta is not filled with cheeses or meats. Stay away from pasta and Italian dishes that have cream sauces or butter. The sauces that are listed as marinara (made with tomatoes, onions, and garlic) and marsala (made with wine) are both tasty and low-fat. Linguini with clam sauce, either red or white, is an Italian low-fat speciality, as is pasta primavera. If pasta is not appealing to you, many Italian dishes are prepared with chicken or fish. Choose an item that is simply prepared and, again, avoid selections that use cheeses and creams.

Chinese Food

There are many selections on the menu at Chinese restaurants that make good low-fat choices. Dishes that are steamed or lightly stir-fried in vegetable oil can be excellent healthy-heart meals. This is particularly true if it is a vegetable, chicken, or seafood selection. Ask that sauces and soy be served on the side. That way you can add just a small amount or none at all, depending on your taste.

The menu at most Chinese restaurants offers you a variety of low-fat, low cholesterol choices, but it is not without pitfalls. There are items you should avoid or limit when eating Chinese food. Avoid the Egg Foo Young and all items served in Lobster Sauce. Both of these selections are made with egg yolks. Main dishes that are deep fried should also be avoided. However, it is more likely that items in a Chinese restaurant will be stir-fried rather than deep-fried. Steamed rice is a better selection than fried rice, which generally contains eggs and may be fried in butter. Ask the server if you have any questions about the preparation. Noodles should be limited. Some soups should be limited due to the addition of noodles, while others should be avoided due to the eggs used in the preparation.

The meat served in Hunan and Szechuan style Chinese cooking is first fried in hot oil and then prepared. For this reason it is best to eliminate these types of foods when adhering to a low-fat food plan. As you have learned, chicken and fish or seafood dishes are generally better low-fat choices than beef or pork.

Japanese Fare

Japanese food, for the most part, is low in cholesterol and saturated fats. The dishes that are listed as "yaki-mono" are good choices for your low cholesterol diet as those are items that have been broiled. The sashimi (raw fish) and sushi (raw fish and rice) are both superb low-cholesterol, low-fat choices. Many traditional Japanese dishes feature vegetables and/or tofu, which is a soybean curd protein that does not contain cholesterol. By and large, Japanese foods, with the exception of tempura, which is prepared by deep frying, are good when following a low cholesterol diet.

Mexican Food

There are many choices for the person interested in limiting cholesterol and saturated fat when eating Mexican. Most items on the menu will fit into a low-fat diet, with the exception of tortilla chips and refried beans. These are both fried in lard and therefore contain large amounts of saturated fat and cholesterol. With these exceptions, there is a whole menu of low-fat vegetable, bean (not refried), chicken, and fish dishes from which to choose. Burritos are made with flour tortillas that are not made with lard and are not fried and would be a good choice. Ask that sour cream, dressings, guacamole, and cheese be served on the side so that you can control their use or eliminate them completely if you choose. So if Mexican suits your taste, there is plenty to choose from without adding fat to your diet.

French Cuisine

Yes, you can eat at French restaurants and still adhere to your low cholesterol, low-fat diet. Probably the most important guideline to remember when eating French cuisine is "make it simply delicious". This means good food with simple preparation. There are many French dishes that are wonderful blends of herbs and spices used in baking or broiling chicken and fish. These would be good low-fat selections. Look for food with simple preparations and the creative use of herbs when making selections at a French restaurant. Menu items that have been broiled with wine are often very tasty, low-fat selections. French cooking is frequently synonymous with sauces and creams. This is just the thing you will want to avoid. The sauces that are used in French cuisine are made with egg yolks, milk, and butter. For example, hollandaise is made with egg yolks and butter, bechamel with milk and butter, bearnaise with egg yolks, and mousseline with egg yolks, butter, and heavy cream. Dishes that are listed as *"nouvelle cuisine"* or *"nouvelle sauces"* may have reduced calorie content and are generally lighter because flour has been eliminated or reduced in the preparation, but they contain saturated fats and cholesterol. For this reason the nouvelle selections would not be wise heart-smart choices.

If a dish is prepared in an acceptable way and the sauce is added after cooking, you may be able to have the sauce held and the dish served without garnish. If you have any questions about the preparation of a dish you are considering, ask your server how it is prepared. Stay away from menu items that are described as au gratin. They will be served with cheese and butter topping.

For dessert you are probably wisest to stay with a fresh fruit selection or a refreshing sorbet. Do not be tempted by the heavy creams and pastries that are usually displayed in French restaurants. Remember, they will only lead to blocking your arteries.

French eating is possible on a low cholesterol, low-fat diet, but it will take some planning and thought on your part. Enjoy your meal, be good to your heart, and keep it simply delicious!

11 Cooking Tips to Lower Saturated Fat and Cholesterol

Now that you know the differences in the types of fats including which ones are good for you, let's put that knowledge to practical use in your own kitchen. Once again, a major consideration is that you must first be a smart shopper and bring food products into the home that are low-fat. With the right ingredients and some modification in your recipes, you can serve delicious heart-smart meals.

We will start our modifications with meats since they are high in saturated fat. In selecting meats, remember that turkey, chicken, and fish have the lowest content of saturated fat. You can often use turkey or chicken in place of beef or pork. For instance, if the recipe calls for ground beef, you can use ground turkey with the same results and less fat. (See recipes included in this chapter.) You should use beef, pork, lamb, or veal no more than two to three times a week. When you do use beef or pork, start with a lean cut; that is, with little marbling and without visible fat. Even lean cuts of meat do contain saturated fat, so it is important to prepare the meat in a way that will minimize the fat. Do not fry meats. Frying adds saturated fat and, additionally, allows the meat to absorb its own fat that could be removed with another cooking method. If your recipe calls for the meat to be browned, place it under the broiler instead of frying. Use a rack to broil, roast, or bake. This allows the fat to drain and, therefore, less is absorbed into the meat. Use low temperatures to roast (250-350 degrees), because slow roasting will allow more fat to cook out of the meat. High temperatures tend to seal, and the fat is then retained. Baste frequently to keep your meat moist while cooking at low temperatures. When you baste, use wine, oil-based marinades, or fruit juices and not the meat drippings, which are saturated fat. Do not flour or bread meats prior to roasting or browning. This also seals the meat and thus retains the fat. Once again, frequent basting can eliminate the potential problem of dry meat. If you remember these tips for selection and preparation, the meats you eat will be lower in saturated fat and still have all of the flavor and great taste you want.

Chicken and turkey are excellent meat substitutes. However, certain processing procedures can change these low-fat meats into highly saturated fat foods. Self basting turkeys are one of the worst offenders. These turkeys are prepared by injecting fat and/or butter under the skin. This causes the turkey to roast in fat, and the fat to be absorbed into the meat. If you buy a fresh or fresh frozen turkey and roast it on a rack, basting it frequently with wines or fruit juice, the turkey will be more delicious and more nutritious. Another example of a perfectly good low-fat source that becomes highly saturated is breaded chicken or turkey products. Many of the breaded foods contain palm and/or coconut oil in the breading along with partially hydrogenated fats. These substances in the breading add unnecessary fats and calories to your otherwise low-fat food. We have also just discussed that breading tends to hold the fats in the meat during the cooking process instead of allowing them to drain away. This information on the breading also holds true for fish products.

You can prepare delicious soups, stews, and gravies with reduced saturated fat by removing the fat from the meat juices. This can be done by cooking the meats a day ahead of time. Then refrigerate the meat in its juices overnight and the fat will harden on the top. If you do not have time to prepare the day before, just put the juices in the freezer or add an ice cube. These methods will also harden the fat for easy removal. Once the fat has hardened, simply remove it from the top of the juices and prepare the dish as directed. You will find that gravies, soups, and stews have a richer flavor when they are prepared in this way.

MEATS AND FISH

Foods to Use	Turkey and chicken without the skin
	Fresh or fresh frozen fish
	Canned fish packed in water
Use in Moderation	Lean cuts beef, veal, and lamb
	Shellfish (shrimp, lobster, crabs, and oysters)
Foods to Avoid	Marbled beef
	Pork (bacon, sausage, pork products)
	Processed meats (hot dogs)
	Luncheon meats
	Fatty fowl (duck, goose)
	Organ meats (liver, kidney, brains)
	Fish canned in oil
	Self basting turkeys, breaded fish and poultry products

DAIRY PRODUCTS CAN BE
LOW IN SATURATED FAT

As you remember from the beginning chapters, dairy products are another major source of cholesterol and saturated fat. This is true because the dairy products are made from an animal source. You know that meat from a cow (beef and veal) is high in saturated fat, so it would logically follow that dairy products that are made from this same source would also be high in saturated fat. Through certain processing, the saturated fat content of dairy products can be reduced. If you learn how to substitute low-fat dairy products for the high-fat products that you are currently using, you can significantly lower your saturated fat intake. Most dairy products have a low-fat substitute available. The labeling of dairy foods is fairly straightforward and easy to interpret. Milk is the easiest example of this high- and low-fat content to illustrate. Milk that is labeled 1% has half of the saturated butter fat of the product that is labeled 2%, and 1/2% or .5% has half of the fat content of the 1% milk. Looking at those labels, it is clear to see that the 1/2% or .5% milk has the lowest butter fat content and would therefore be the best choice. Always use the .5% or skim milk to give you the lowest saturated fat content. This means that the milk is 99.5% fat free.

Another dairy product that has a high saturated fat content is cheese. Look for cheeses that are made with skim milk rather than whole milk. Some examples of skim milk cheeses are mozzarella, farmer's, and low-fat uncreamed cottage. Some cheeses that are made with skim milk have cream added to them. For this reason it is important to check the package label of cheese products even if they say, "made with skim milk". You don't want a cheese that has additional saturated fat added in the form of cream. You an be a smart shopper if you take time to read those package labels. As we said in Chapter 5, the initial label reading will take time. But once you find a product that is low-fat and tastes good to you, shopping will be easier. Most people stick with the same product for years once they find what they want.

There are other dairy products that have low-fat substitutes available. You can use evaporated skim milk or liquid non-dairy creamer in place of heavy cream. Just substitute equal amounts. That means if your recipe calls for one cup of heavy cream, you can use one cup of evaporated skim milk with the same results. Instead of high-fat yogurt, sometimes labeled as creamy, use part skim yogurt. You can also use low-fat yogurt in recipes that call for sour cream. If you do not like the taste of low-fat yogurt on baked potatoes or as a sour cream dressing, you can use the mock sour cream recipe found in this chapter. There are some imitation sour cream products commercially available, but many of them contain palm and/or coconut oil. (Remember that palm and coconut oils are saturated fats.)

In talking about dairy products we should also mention eggs. You know that egg yolks contain about 275 mg. of cholesterol. You should limit your intake of egg yolks to 3 yolks per week. Most people are able to limit their intake of whole eggs as a part of a meal to 3 a week. But what about all the cooking that requires eggs? You can use either an egg substitute or just the egg whites from whole eggs. If you use an egg substitute, be sure that you read the label, as some do contain cholesterol. There are other substitutes that contain no cholesterol, and these would be a better choice. The egg substitutes have whole egg equivalents listed on their labels. For example, 1/4 cup of egg substitute may equal one whole egg. In a recipe that called for one egg you would then use 1/4 cup of that particular substitute. If you use egg whites in place of the whole egg, it is a two to one substitution. That is, one whole egg is equal to two egg whites in a recipe. If you use egg whites, you will be missing the yellow coloring that the yolk provides. The yellow may not be important if it is in a cake batter or a sauce. However, there are times when the yellow will be missed, as in scrambled eggs for example. To get that yellow color that is missing from the whites, you may want to add one drop of food coloring for every two egg whites. Be careful; too much color makes it look like you are eating fluorescent scrambled eggs. The food coloring doesn't change the flavor, but appearance of food is probably just as important as taste.

Ice cream is a dairy product that most of us love and certainly enjoy from time to time. Ice cream has a high butter fat content (in some products as much as 45–50%) and, therefore, a high saturated fat content. There are low-fat substitutes that are available. These products are labeled as Ice Milk. Once again, some ice milks are made with palm and/or coconut oil and are **not** low-fat choices. Read the labels and find the low-fat ice milk that suits your taste.

While dairy products are high in saturated fat and cholesterol because they are from animal sources, there are many low-fat substitutes available. Use the substitutes listed below to help you make good low-fat choices. In that way, you can continue to enjoy all of the good taste of dairy products without the harmful effects of saturated fat and cholesterol.

USE	AVOID
Skim milk or .5% milk	Whole milk
Low-fat cheeses	Whole milk cheese
Low-fat or partial skim yogurt	Creamy or high-fat yogurt

USE	AVOID
Evaporated skim milk	Heavy cream
Liquid non-dairy creamer	
Low-fat yogurt or	Sour cream
mock sour cream or	
imitation sour cream	
Egg whites or	Whole eggs
egg substitute	
Ice milk	Ice cream

COOKING WITH FATS AND OILS

The majority of saturated fat that you ingest comes from three categories of foods. These are meat and meat products, dairy foods, and fats. We have just examined meat and dairy products and their appropriate low saturated fat substitutions, so now we will tackle the fat category. To determine which fats are highly saturated you will want to keep in mind the two rules that you learned in Chapter 3. If it comes from an animal source or is solid at room temperature, it contains saturated fat. Again, we stress that the exceptions are palm and coconut oils. Both are high in saturated fat even though they are from a vegetable source and are liquid. With that in mind, look at your eating habits and examine your recipes for ways to decrease your saturated fat intake and increase the unsaturated fats. Your best substitutions will be made by choosing vegetable products that contain no palm or coconut oil and are liquid.

What kind of fats do you use that are highly saturated? Any fat that comes from an animal source is certainly a saturated fat. That includes butter, lard, bacon drippings, chicken fat, cream sauces, and drippings from all meat preparation. Secondly, any fat product that is solid at room temperature contains saturated fat. Some examples of that would be shortening and margarine. You can substitute any of these with a good low saturated fat choice. Using a liquid vegetable oil would be an excellent low saturated fat choice, since it is both liquid and vegetable in origin. Safflower oil has the lowest amount of saturated and the highest polyunsaturated fat available, so it would be a good choice as a substitute. (See Chapter 3.) Some people find the taste of safflower oil bitter and do not choose to use it. Give safflower oil a try because it is the highest polyunsaturated and low in saturated fat, but if it is not to your liking, there are many other vegetable oils available. An excellent alternative is canola oil, also called rapeseed oil. Canola oil is very low in saturated fats, but instead of high amounts of polyunsaturated fats, it contains high levels of monounsaturated fats. Included in these monounsaturated fats are the omega 3 type (See Chapter 3). You may have to test several different products to find the one that suits your particular taste.

You will find that there are times when a liquid is inappropriate as a substitute for the saturated fat. For example, you wouldn't want to put oil on toast. In these cases you will want to use a low saturated fat in a solid form, like margarine. Margarine is made from a vegetable, usually corn, but it is solid at room temperature. It meets one of the two criteria for a good low saturated fat, but not both. This means that margarine has less saturated fat than butter, but more than vegetable oil. Once you decide to use a margarine, you must then decide if it should be stick or soft. Since margarine is from vegetable, the only other consideration is the solidity factor. Stick margarine is harder so it contains more saturated fat. Your best margarine choice, therefore, is soft margarine. It's a little like the old saying: "Good, better, best, don't let it rest, till your good is better, and your better is best." Oil is the best fat choice you can make, as long as it is not palm or coconut oil. Soft margarine is the better choice, and stick is a good choice. Whenever you can, use oil for your cooking or in recipes. If oil is not appropriate, then soft margarine would be the next best choice. If you can not use soft margarine, then stick would be better than butter or some other animal saturated fat. It will take some experimenting to find which oil and soft margarine taste better to you. But isn't it nice to have so many low saturated choices available to you? You will find some recipes in this chapter that have been adapted and use low saturated fat substitutes. To make it easy for you to do this with your own family's favorite recipes, use the conversion guide on page 112.

The final source of saturated fat we would like to discuss is chocolate or any form of cocoa butter. Both cocoa butter and the chocolate that is made from it contain saturated fat. Cocoa powder and carob contain saturated fat, but in very reduced amounts in comparison to chocolate. Look for chocolate products that are made from either cocoa powder or carob. Chocolate can be replaced in many of your recipes by substituting cocoa powder and polyunsaturated oil. One ounce of baking chocolate contains 8.4 grams of saturated fat. By comparison 3 tablespoons of cocoa powder combined with 1 tablespoon of vegetable oil contains .8 grams of saturated fat, and produces the same results.

You have learned how to make good, low-fat substitutions in your buying and eating habits. Making changes in your eating patterns is not something you can do overnight. The saying—every little bit helps—can be applied to your efforts to reduce saturated fat from your diet. Whenever you choose a low saturated fat product, you are helping to reduce the amount of fat in your coronary arteries. The war against heart disease is fought with each food choice you make. Every little step helps, and pretty soon you have a lot of little steps making big strides in keeping your heart healthy. Be patient with yourself in making these substitutions and changes. Above all, keep trying!

Use the following substitutions of oils for fats:

USE	IN PLACE OF
7/8 cup of polyunsaturated oil or 1 cup soft or tub margarine or 1 cup (2 sticks) margarine	1 cup butter
3 tablespoons cocoa powder plus 1 tablespoon polyunsaturated oil	1 ounce baking chocolate
polyunsaturated oil or soft margarine or stick margarine	shortening, lard, bacon fat, chicken fat, or meat drippings

DELICIOUS LOW-FAT RECIPES

These recipes are included in this book to give you examples of how to begin thinking about altering your current recipes to make them good low-fat selections. Many low-cholesterol recipe books are currently on the market to help you add to the meals you are now preparing. We think it is a more beneficial approach to learn to adapt the recipes you use and like. For that reason we have selected some recipes which represent different types of dishes that you may already be serving. However, these recipes are prepared in a low cholesterol, low saturated fat way.

Soups

EGG DROP SOUP

Traditionally, Egg Drop Soup is made with whole eggs and occasionally additional egg yolks. Our Egg Drop Soup uses egg substitute and still delivers all of the rich full taste of the traditional soup, without cholesterol.

4 cups of water	1/4 teaspoon tarragon
4 cubes low sodium chicken bouillon	1/4 cup egg substitute
3 tablespoons cornstarch	

Bring 3½ cups water to boil in a medium sauce pan. Add chicken bouillon to boiling water. Stir until bouillon is dissolved. Combine the cornstarch with the remaining 1/2 cup water. Add cornstarch to the dissolved bouillon, stirring constantly. Mix in tarragon. Cook over medium heat until thickened and boiling. Continue to cook for one minute longer. Reduce heat to low and slowly add egg substitute. Add egg substitute in a thin stream. *Do not* stir while adding the egg substitute. Cook for about one minute. Stir once before removing from heat. Serves 6

HALIBUT BISQUE

Bisques are usually made with heavy creams, milk, and butter, which are high cholesterol and saturated fat foods. You can enjoy all of the flavor of a bisque without the fat and cholesterol containing ingredients by using substitutes. Try our version of Halibut Bisque, a delicious, creamy creation.

2 tablespoons onion, chopped	dash salt
2 tablespoons chopped celery	1/4 teaspoon paprika
1/4 cup soft margarine, melted	dash pepper
2 tablespoons flour	1 quart skim milk
nutmeg	3/4 pound cooked flaky halibut

Cook onion and celery in margarine in pot until tender and onions are clear. Blend in flour and all seasonings, except nutmeg. Stir in milk gradually. Cook until thickened, stirring constantly. Add halibut. Cook over low heat for 30–45 minutes, stirring occasionally. Garnish with nutmeg. Serves 6

CHICKEN STOCK

There are many recipes for preparing chicken stock. This one is rich in flavor and low in fats and salt. This easy chicken stock can be prepared in quantity and then frozen for uses in different ways. You will find many ways of using the chicken stock in recipes. (One example follows.)

5 pounds skinless chicken	1/3 cup diced carrots
3 quarts water	1/3 cup diced onion
2 sprigs parsley	1/2 cup diced celery
1/4 teaspoon thyme	dash salt
1 crumbled bay leaf	fresh ground pepper

In a pot combine chicken and water. Bring to a slow boil. Skim any fat off top of water after boil. Add all remaining ingredients. Cover and simmer over low heat. Cook approximately 3 1/2 hours. Skim fat from top prior to cooling. Yield: 2 1/2 quarts.

Many low-fat ingredients may be added to the basic chicken stock to create some wonderful low-fat soups. Here's an example:

MATZO BALL SOUP

These low-fat, low cholesterol matzo balls are light and fluffy without the eggs and chicken fat generally associated with them. Add these matzo balls to your chicken stock for a delicious hot soup.

1/4 cup cold water	1 egg white
2 tablespoons soft margarine	1/2 cup matzo meal
1/4 cup egg substitute	1/4 teaspoon salt
6 cups chicken stock	

Combine water, margarine, egg substitute, and egg white in a bowl. Add matzo meal, stirring constantly. Blend in salt. Cover and refrigerate for 30 minutes. Warm chicken stock over medium heat. Take cooled matzo mixture from refrigerator and drop rounded teaspoonfuls on top of just boiling chicken stock. Cover and cook at a slow boil for 20 minutes. Serve piping hot. Serves 4

Salad Dressings

As you have learned, salads are good low-fat, low cholesterol additions to a meal. However, the dressings that are used to top these good healthful foods are many times less than desirable low-fat choices. Here are some dressings you can make that are delicious, easy to make, and excellent cholesterol-conscious accompaniments to any salad. You may also want to take your own low cholesterol, low-fat dressings in a small container when you are dining out.

MAYONNAISE

1/3 cup egg substitute	dash ground pepper
1 teaspoon dry mustard	2 tablespoons vinegar
1/4 teaspoon onion powder	1 cup vegetable oil
1/4 teaspoon paprika	

Combine first six ingredients and one half cup of vegetable oil in blender or food processor. Cover and blend until just mixed. (Pulse mode on many food processors works quite well for this mixing.) Put blender on medium speed, or with food processor on, slowly add remaining 1/2 cup vegetable oil in a thin stream. Continue to blend until oil is completely absorbed in mixture. Use a rubber spatula to keep ingredients moving during mixing if they adhere to side. Cover and refrigerate. Makes 1 1/2 cups

MOCK SOUR CREAM

2 tablespoons skim milk	1 cup low-fat ricotta cheese
1 tablespoon lemon juice	

Place all ingredients in a blender and mix on medium high until smooth and creamy. This recipe may also be prepared in a food processor if you desire.

POPPY SEED DRESSING

1/2 cup mayonnaise (see above)	1 tablespoon poppy seeds

2 tablespoons sugar   1 tablespoon lemon
                                               juice

Combine all ingredients in a bowl and mix thoroughly.
Cover and chill at least one hour. Makes 1 cup

RUSSIAN DRESSING

2 1/2 cups mayonnaise   6 tablespoons catsup
   (see above)

1 tablespoon Worcester-   1 tablespoon minced
   shire sauce   onion

Combine all ingredients in a bowl and beat with mixer
on low speed until completely blended, approximately 5
minutes. Cover and chill before serving. Makes 3 cups

FRUITY DRESSING

2 1/4 teaspoons sugar   3/4 cup pineapple juice

3/4 teaspoon salt   3/4 cup lemon juice

1 cup oil

Combine sugar and salt in a bowl. Slowly add oil and
fruit juices. Mix thoroughly in blender or food processor.
Cover and chill for at least 1 hour before serving. Makes
2 1/2 cups

CREAMY GARLIC DRESSING

1 cup mock sour cream   dash salt
   (see above)

1/2 teaspoon sugar   dash pepper

1 teaspoon garlic powder   1/2 teaspoon paprika

1/2 teaspoon dry mustard

Combine all ingredients in a bowl and mix thoroughly. Cover and chill before serving. Makes 1 cup

Chicken and Turkey Dishes

There are several thousand recipes that contain chicken and turkey. The recipes that follow in this section are to give you an idea of the tremendous variety of dishes that can be prepared using chicken and turkey, some of which you may only associate with beef or pork. Once again the important consideration in this section is for you to adapt your recipes and make them good low cholesterol, low-fat meals.

CRISPY SOUTHERN CHICKEN

Usually southern chicken is coated with the skin on and fried in shortening. This recipe gives you that crispy coating and juicy taste you love without the fat and cholesterol.

3 pounds skinless chicken   1 cup skim milk

1 cup cornflake crumbs   salt, pepper to taste

3 tablespoons oil

Preheat oven to 400° F. Remove the skin from the chicken and pat dry. Season chicken to taste. Dip chicken in milk and shake off excess. Thoroughly coat chicken with the cornflake crumbs. Let chicken sit to allow coating to adhere to chicken before placing in baking dish. Oil baking dish. Place chicken in dish. Bake for 45 min. at 400°F. Chicken will be tender, juicy, and crispy. Serves 4

CHICKEN KABOBS

6 chicken breasts, skinless and deboned

12 small cherry tomatoes

2 medium onions, quartered

12 mushrooms

Cut chicken breasts into pieces for the skewers. Alternate chicken, tomatoes, onions, and mushrooms on skewer. Place skewers in marinade for about 30 minutes.

CHICKEN KABOB MARINADE

1/2 cup oil	1/8 teaspoon pepper
1 clove garlic, crushed	1/8 teaspoon lemon
1 tablespoon vinegar	juice

Mix all ingredients together. Place marinade in a glass baking dish. *Do not use a metal pan.* Place chicken kabobs in marinade. After kabobs have marinated for 30 minutes, cook either under broiler on on grill. Cook 10 to 15 minutes, turning and basting with marinade at least twice during cooking. Serve warm marinade over kabobs. Serves 6

GROUND TURKEY CHILI

Once you try this hearty turkey chili you will be convinced that low-fat meals can be better than the old high saturated fat variety.

1/4 cup chopped onion	1/4 teaspoon oregano
1 clove garlic	1/4 teaspoon paprika
5 tablespoons oil	2-15 oz. cans tomato
1 pound ground turkey	sauce
3 tablespoons chili powder	1-6 oz. can tomato
	paste
	2-15 oz. cans kidney
	beans

In a medium skillet, saute onion and garlic in 1 tablespoon oil until tender and clear. Add remaining oil and warm over medium heat. Do not overheat oil. Add ground turkey to oil, onion and garlic mixture. Cook turkey slowly and break up ground turkey frequently. If you are not used to cooking with ground turkey, it becomes a white gray color as it cooks. It does not brown as ground beef does. In a large pot combine tomato sauce, kidney beans, and tomato paste. Add chili powder, oregano, and paprika to tomato sauce mixture. Add ground turkey mixture to tomato sauce and cook over low heat for 1 1/2 to 2 hours, stirring occasionally. Serve topped with chopped onions and tomatoes. Serves 8

Ground turkey can be used in most recipes that call for ground beef. Try it in your meatballs or meat sauce and spaghetti. Turkey meatloaf is a hearty delicious meal. Use the same recipes that you have for years. Just substitute good low-fat meats, oils, and margarines for the beef, pork, lard, shortening, and butter. You will find that most of your favorite dishes are completely adaptable and are lighter and full of flavor.

TURKEY MARSALA

This is an elegant meal that will impress your friends and relatives at any dinner party. It is easy to prepare and quite inexpensive, but the results are magnificent.

2 pounds turkey cutlet	1/2 cup Marsala
1/2 cup flour	1 tablespoon soft margarine
4 tablespoons oil	3 tablespoons beef consommé
1 tablespoon soft margarine	1/2 pound mushrooms

Pound turkey cutlets between two pieces of waxed paper until 1/4 inch thick. Dredge cutlet through flour. Do not dry cutlet prior to flouring. Shake off excess flour. In skillet, heat oil and margarine until hot. Margarine will begin to bubble. Add cutlet to hot oil mixture; turn once when edges become white. Continue to cook until cutlet becomes lightly browned. Do not overcook cutlets as they will become tough. Cutlets cook very quickly, so watch carefully. When cutlets are browned, remove from oil. To the oil and margarine in the pan, add Marsala, consommé, margarine, and mushrooms over medium heat. If the sauce is too thin, you may add 1 tablespoon of flour to sauce to thicken. Add flour slowly, stirring constantly. When sauce is smooth, add cutlets; stir and coat until covered. Serve immediately. Serves 8

Desserts

The following are some examples of good heart-smart desserts you can make at home. These recipes are easy and delicious. You don't have to deprive yourself of dessert just because you are on a low-fat food plan. There are many low-fat cookbooks on the market if you are interested in adding to your recipes. Remember, you may be able to make substitutions and changes in the recipes you currently use.

LOW-FAT WHIPPED CREAM SUBSTITUTE

1 teaspoon Knox gelatin

3 tablespoons boiling water

4 tablespoons sugar

1/2 cup ice water

3/4 cup nonfat dry milk (which contains no palm or coconut oil)

3 tablespoons corn or soybean/cottonseed oil

Place gelatin in boiling water and dissolve completely, stirring continuously. Allow the gelatin mixture to cool to room temperature. While gelatin mixture is cooling, put a deep narrow mixing bowl into the freezer for approximately 15 minutes. Mix nonfat dry milk and ice water in the bowl from freezer and blend together at high speed. Using high speed, slowly add sugar to dry milk mixture. When the dry milk, water, and sugar mixture takes on a creamy appearance, begin to add the room temperature gelatin mixture. After completely blending the gelatin mixture at high speed, slowly drizzle the oil into the mixture. Mix all ingredients at high speed. Freeze overnight and then place in refrigerator for at least four hours prior to serving.

STRAWBERRY CREAM PIE

This cool and refreshing low-fat dessert will delight your family and impress your friends.

1 pint fresh strawberries
1 package (4 serving size) instant vanilla pudding
1 cup mock sour cream
1/4 cup skim milk
2 teaspoons grated orange or lemon peel
3 1/2 cups Low-fat Whipped Cream Substitute
graham cracker pie crust

Hull berries and set aside. Combine instant pudding, mock sour cream, milk, and citrus peel. When combined, add 2 cups topping. Beat with wire wisk until well blended, about 1 minute. Spoon half of filling into pie crust. Arrange berries on filling and press down. Add remaining half of filling. Freeze for 1 hour or chill for 3 hours before serving. Garnish with additional strawberries and whipped topping. Makes one 9-inch pie

PIE CRUST

2 cups flour

1 teaspoon salt

1/2 cup oil

1/4 cup + 1 tablespoon cold water

In a large mixing bowl, sift flour and salt. Mix oil and water together until foamy and add to flour and salt mixture. Blend well. Divide into two portions. Roll out crust on waxed paper. Place one rolled out dough into pie pan. After adding pie filling, use the second portion of the dough for the top crust. Bake in preheated oven at 425° until done. Yields: two pie crusts

FUDGY BROWNIES

1/2 cup oil

3 egg whites

3/4 cup sugar

1 teaspoon vanilla
   extract

1/2 teaspoon baking
   powder

1/2 cup chopped
   walnuts (optional)

1/2 cup all purpose flour

6 tablespoons unsweetened carob powder *or*
   Nestles Quick

Preheat oven to 350° F. Oil bottom and sides of 8-inch baking dish. Combine oil, egg whites, sugar, and vanilla in a large mixing bowl. Blend in flour, carob, or Quick, and baking powder. Do not sift flour. Stir in nuts if desired. Pour batter into prepared baking dish. Bake 15 to 20 minutes or until a toothpick inserted into center comes out clean. Cool completely before cutting into squares. Makes 16 brownies

Appendix 1

Cholesterol Lowering Diet Recommended for All Americans Over the Age of Two

Less than 30% Fat
(Total Daily Calories)

{
Less than 10% from
Saturated Fat

10%–15% from
Monounsaturated Fat

Up to 10% from
Polyunsaturated Fat
}

Less Than 300 mg. of Cholesterol a Day
50–60% *Total Daily Calories from Carbohydrates*
(primarily complex carbohydrates)

Up to 20% Daily Calories from Protein

Total Calories to Achieve and Maintain Ideal Weight

Appendix 2

Saturated Fat, Cholesterol, Total Fat, and Calorie Content of Foods

When controlling cholesterol, it is essential to know the saturated fat and cholesterol content of foods. The following charts list the saturated fat, cholesterol, total fat, percent of calories from fat and total calories for many foods. These tables are arranged into particular types of food to make it easier to find a certain item.

MEATS

Meats are a major source of saturated fat and cholesterol in the diet. The following list includes various cuts of beef, lamb, pork, and veal. Use lean cuts of meat and prepare utilizing the suggestions in Chapter 11 to reduce the saturated fat content.

Product (3½ Ounces, Cooked)*	Saturated Fatty Acids (Grams)	Cholesterol (Milligrams)	Fat[1] (Grams)	Calories From Fat[2] (%)	Total Calories
Beef					
Kidneys, Simmered[3]	1.1	387	3.4	21	144
Liver, Braised[3]	1.9	389	4.9	27	161
Round, top round, lean only, broiled	2.2	84	6.2	29	191
Round, eye of round, lean only, broasted	2.5	69	6.5	32	183
Round, tip round, lean only, roasted	2.8	81	7.5	36	190
Round, full cut, lean only, choice, broiled	2.9	82	8.0	37	194
Round, bottom round, lean only, braised	3.4	96	9.7	39	222
Short loin, top loin, lean only, broiled	3.6	76	8.9	40	203
Wedge-bone sirloin, lean only, broiled	3.6	89	8.7	38	208
Short loin, tenderloin, lean only broiled	3.6	84	9.3	41	204
Chuck, arm pot roast, lean only, braised	3.8	101	10.0	39	231
Short loin, T-bone steak, lean only, choice, broiled	4.2	80	10.4	44	214

*3½ ozs = 100 grams (approximately)

[1]Total fat = saturated fatty acids plus monounsaturated fatty acids plus polyunsaturated fatty acids.

[2]Percent calories from fat = (total fat calories divided by total calories) multiplied by 100; total fat calories = total fat (grams) multiplied by 9.

[3]Liver and most organ meals are low in fat, but high in cholesterol. If you are eating to lower your blood cholesterol, you should consider your total cholesterol intake before selecting an organ meat.

Product (3½ Ounces, Cooked)*	Saturated Fatty Acids (Grams)	Cholesterol (Milligrams)	Fat[1] (Grams)	Calories From Fat[2] (%)	Total Calories
Short loin, porterhouse steak, lean only, choice, broiled	4.3	80	10.8	45	218
Brisket, whole, lean only, braised	4.6	93	12.8	48	241
Rib eye, small end (ribs 10-12), lean only, choice, broiled	4.9	80	11.6	47	225
Rib, whoel (ribs 6-12), lean only, roasted	5.8	81	13.8	52	240
Flank, lean only, choice, braised	5.9	71	13.8	51	244
Rib, large ends (ribs 6-9), lean only, broiled	6.1	82	14.2	55	233
Chuck, blade roast, lean only, braised	6.2	106	15.3	51	270
Corned beef, cured, brisket, cooked	6.3	98	19.0	68	251
Flank, lean and fat, choice, braised	6.6	72	15.5	54	257
Ground, lean, broiled medium	7.2	87	18.5	61	272
Round, full cut, lean and fat, choice, braised	7.3	84	18.2	60	274
Rib, short ribs, lean and fat, choice, braised	7.7	93	18.1	55	295
Salami, cured, cooked, smoked, 3-4 slices	9.0	65	20.7	71	262
Short loin, T-bone steak, lean and fat, choice, broiled	10.2	84	24.6	68	324
Chuck, arm pot roast, lean and fat, braised	10.7	99	26.0	67	350

Product (3½ Ounces, Cooked)*	Saturated Fatty Acids (Grams)	Cholesterol (Milligrams)	Fat[1] (Grams)	Calories From Fat[2] (%)	Total Calories
Sausage, cured, cooked, smoked, about 2	11.4	67	26.9	78	312
Bologna, cured, 3-4 slices	12.1	58	28.5	82	312
Frankfurter, cured, about 2	12.0	61	28.5	82	315
Lamb					
Leg, lean only, roasted	3.0	89	8.2	39	191
Loin chop, lean only, broiled	4.1	94	9.4	39	215
Rib, lean only, roasted	5.7	88	12.3	48	232
Arm chop, lean only, braised	6.0	122	14.6	47	279
Rib, lean and fat, roasted	14.2	90	30.6	75	368
Pork					
Cured, ham steak, boneless, extra lean, unheated	1.4	45	4.2	31	122
Liver, braised[3]	1.4	355	4.4	24	165
Kidneys, braised[3]	1.5	480	4.7	28	151
Fresh, loin, tenderloin, lean only, roasted	2.4	48	7.0	37	170
Cured, shoulder, arm picnic, lean only, roasted	2.4	48	7.0	37	170
Cured, ham, boneless, regular, roasted	3.1	59	9.0	46	178
Fresh, leg (ham), shank half, lean only, roasted	3.6	92	10.5	44	215
Fresh, leg (ham), rump half, lean only, roasted	3.7	96	10.7	43	221

Product (3½ Ounces, Cooked)*	Saturated Fatty Acids (Grams)	Cholesterol (Milligrams)	Fat[1] (Grams)	Calories From Fat[2] (%)	Total Calories
Fresh loin, center loin, sirloin, lean only, roasted	4.5	90	13.2	50	236
Fresh, loin, center rib, lean only, roasted	4.8	79	13.8	51	245
Fresh, loin, top loin, lean only, roasted	4.8	79	13.8	51	245
Fresh, shoulder, blade, Boston, lean only, roasted	5.8	98	16.8	59	256
Fresh, loin, blade, lean only, roasted	6.6	89	19.3	62	279
Fresh, loin, sirloin, lean and fat, roasted	7.4	91	20.4	63	291
Cured, shoulder, arm picnic, lean and fat, roasted	7.7	58	21.4	69	280
Fresh, loin, center loin, lean and fat, roasted	7.9	91	21.8	64	305
Cured, shoulder, blade roll, lean and fat, roasted	8.4	67	23.5	74	287
Fresh, Italian sausage, cooked	9.0	78	25.7	72	323
Fresh, bratwurst, cooked	9.3	60	25.9	77	301
Fresh, chitterlings, cooked	10.1	143	28.8	86	303
Cured, liver sausage, liverwurst	10.6	158	28.5	79	326
Cured, smoked link sausage, grilled	11.3	68	31.8	74	389
Fresh, spareribs, lean and fat, braised	11.8	121	30.3	69	397
Cured, salami, dry or hard	11.9	—	33.7	75	407

— = information not available in the sources used.

Product (3½ Ounces, Cooked)*	Saturated Fatty Acids (Grams)	Cholesterol (Milligrams)	Fat[1] (Grams)	Calories From Fat[2] (%)	Total Calories
Bacon, fried	17.4	85	49.2	78	576
Veal					
Rump, lean only, roasted	—	128	2.2	13	156
Sirloin, lean only, roasted	—	128	3.2	19	153
Arm steak, lean only, cooked	—	90	5.3	24	200
Loin chop, lean only, cooked	—	90	6.7	29	207
Blade, lean only, cooked	—	90	7.8	33	211
Cutlet, medium fat, braised or broiled	4.8	128	11.0	37	271
Foreshank, medium fat, stewed	—	90	10.4	43	216
Plate, medium fat, stewed	—	90	21.2	63	303
Rib, medium fat, roasted	7.1	128	16.9	70	218
Flank, medium fat, stewed	—	90	32.3	75	390

Sources:

Composition of Foods: Beef Products - Raw • Processed • Prepared, Agricultural Handbook 8-13. United States Department of Agriculture, Human Nutrition Information Service (August 1986)

Composition of Foods: Pork Products - Raw• Processed • Prepared, Agricultural Handbook 8-10. United States Department of Agriculture, Human Nutrition Information Service (August 1983).

Home and Garden Bulletin. Nutritive Value of Foods. No. 72. United States Department of Agriculture. Human Nutrition Information Service (1986).

POULTRY

Poultry is generally lower in saturated fat and cholesterol than most cuts of meat. This is especially true when the skin has been removed. The following table gives saturated fat, cholesterol and calorie content of several selections of chicken and turkey.

Product (3½ Ounces, Cooked)*	Saturated Fatty Acids (Grams)	Cholesterol (Milligrams)	Fat[1] (Grams)	Calories From Fat[2] (%)	Total Calories
Turkey, fryer-roasters, light meat without skin, roasted	0.4	86	1.9	8	140
Chicken, roasters, light meat without skin, roasted	1.1	75	4.1	24	153
Turkey, fryer-roasters, light meat with skin, roasted	1.3	95	4.6	25	164
Chicken, broilers or fryers, light meat without skin, roasted	1.3	85	4.5	24	173
Turkey, fryer-roasters, dark meat without skin, roasted	1.4	112	4.3	24	162
Chicken, stewing, light meat without skin, stewed	2.0	70	8.0	34	213
Turkey roll, light and dark	2.0	55	7.0	42	149

*3½ ozs = 100 grams (approximately)
[1]Total fat = saturated fatty acids plus monounsaturated fatty acids plus polyunsaturated fatty acids.
[2]Percent calories from fat = (total fat calories divided by total calories) multiplied by 100; total fat calories = total fat (grams) multiplied by 9.

Product (3¹/₂ Ounces, Cooked)*	Saturated Fatty Acids (Grams)	Cholesterol (Milligrams)	Fat[1] (Grams)	Calories From Fat[2] (%)	Total Calories
Turkey, fryer-roasters, dark meat with skin, roasted	2.1	117	7.1	35	182
Chicken, roasters, dark meat without skin, roasted	2.4	75	8.8	44	178
Chicken, broilers or fryers, dark meat without skin, roasted	2.7	93	9.7	43	205
Chicken, broilers or fryers, light meat with skin, roasted	3.0	84	10.9	44	222
Chicken, stewing, dark meat without skin, stewed	4.1	95	15.3	53	258
Duck, domesticated, flesh only, roasted	4.2	89	11.2	50	201
Chicken, broilers or fryers, dark meat with skin, roasted	4.4	91	15.8	56	253
Goose, domesticated, flesh only, roasted	4.6	96	12.7	48	238
Turkey bologna, about 3¹/₂ slices	5.1	99	15.2	69	199
Chicken frankfurter, about 2	5.9	107	17.7	70	226

Source:

Composition of Foods: Poultry Products - Raw • Processed • Prepared, Agricultural Handbook 8-5. United States Department of Agriculture, Science and Education Administration (August 1979).

FISH AND SHELLFISH

To help lower cholesterol, you will want to include more fish and shellfish in your diet. Fish and shellfish are lower in saturated fat than meat or poultry. Some shellfish, however, do contain cholesterol and their use should be limited to meet the cholesterol limitations. Omega-3 fatty acids are found in fish and shellfish and have been shown to be beneficial in reducing cholesterol. (See Chapter 3.) This table gives the saturated fat, cholesterol, Omega-3 fatty acids, total fat, calories from fat, and total calorie content of selected fish and shellfish.

Product (3¹/₂ Ounces, Cooked)*	Saturated Fatty Acids (Grams)	Cholesterol (Milligrams)	Omega-3 Fatty Acids (Grams)	Fat[1] (Grams)	Calories From Fat[2] (%)	Total Calories
Finfish						
Haddock, dry heat	0.2	74	0.2	0.9	7	112
Cod, Atlantic, dry heat	0.2	55	0.2	0.9	7	105
Pollock, walleye, dry heat	0.2	96	1.5	1.1	9	113
Perch, mixed species, dry heat	0.2	42	0.3	1.2	9	117
Grouper, mixed species, dry heat	0.3	47	—	1.3	10	118
Whiting, mixed species, dry heat	0.3	84	0.9	1.7	13	115
Snapper, mixed species, dry heat	0.4	47	—	1.7	12	128
Halibut, Atlantic and Pacific, dry heat	0.4	41	0.6	2.9	19	140
Rockfish, Pacific, dry heat	0.5	44	0.5	2.0	15	121
Sea bass, mixed species, dry heat	0.7	53	—	2.5	19	124

*3¹/₂ ozs. = 100 grams (approximately).

[1]Total fat = saturated fatty acids plus monounsaturated fatty acids plus polyunsaturated fatty acids.

[2]Percent calories from fat = (total fat calories divided by total calories) multiplied by 100; total fat calories = total fat (grams) multiplied by 9.

— = Information not available in sources used.

Product (3½ Ounces, Cooked)*	Saturated Fatty Acids (Grams)	Cholesterol (Milligrams)	Omega-3 Fatty Acids (Grams)	Fat[1] (Grams)	Calories From Fat[2] (%)	Total Calories
Trout, rainbow, dry heat	0.8	73	0.9	4.3	26	151
Swordfish, dry heat	1.4	50	1.1	5.1	30	155
Tuna, bluefin, dry heat	1.6	49	—	6.3	31	184
Salmon, sockeye, dry heat	1.9	87	1.3	11.0	46	216
Anchovy, European, canned	2.2	—	2.1	9.7	42	210
Herring, Atlantic, dry heat	2.6	77	2.1	11.5	51	203
Eel, dry heat	3.0	161	0.7	15.0	57	236
Mackerel, Atlantic, dry heat	4.2	75	1.3	17.8	61	262
Pompano, Florida, dry heat	4.5	64	—	12.1	52	211
Crustaceans						
Lobster, northern	0.1	72	0.1	0.6	6	98
Crab, blue, moist heat	0.2	100	0.5	1.8	16	102
Shrimp, mixed species, moist heat	0.3	195	0.3	1.1	10	99
Mollusks						
Whelk, moist heat	0.1	130	—	0.8	3	275
Clam, mixed species, moist heat	0.2	67	0.3	2.0	12	148
Mussel, blue, moist heat	0.9	56	0.8	4.5	23	172
Oyster, Eastern, moist heat	1.3	109	1.0	5.0	33	137

Source:
Composition of Foods: Finfish and Shellfish Products - Raw • Processed • Prepared, Agriculture Handbook 8-15. United States Department of Agriculture (in press).

DAIRY AND EGG PRODUCTS

Dairy products contain both saturated fat and cholesterol. When selecting dairy products choose those with the lowest butterfat content. Egg yolks are a major source of cholesterol. Egg whites or substitutes should be used in place of egg yolks.

Product (3½ Ounces, Cooked)*	Saturated Fatty Acids (Grams)	Cholesterol (Milligrams)	Fat[1] (Grams)	Calories From Fat[2] (%)	Total Calories
Milk (8 ounces)					
Skim milk	0.3	4	0.4	5	86
Buttermilk	1.3	9	2.2	20	99
Low-fat milk, 1% fat	1.6	10	2.6	23	102
Low-fat milk, 2% fat	2.9	18	4.7	35	121
Whole milk, 3.3% fat	5.1	33	8.2	49	150
Yogurt (4 ounces)					
Plain yogurt, low-fat	0.1	2	0.2	3	63
Plain yogurt	2.4	14	3.7	47	70
Cheese					
Cottage cheese, low-fat, 1% fat, 4 oz.	0.7	5	1.2	13	82
Mozzarella, part-skim, 1 oz.	2.9	16	4.5	56	72
Cottage cheese, creamed, 4 oz.	3.2	17	5.1	39	117
Mozzarella, 1 oz.	3.7	22	6.1	69	80
Sour cream, 1 oz.	3.7	12	5.9	87	61
American processed cheese spread, pasteurized, 1 oz.	3.8	16	6.0	66	82

[1]Total fat = saturated fatty acids plus monounsaturated fatty acids plus polyunsaturated fatty acids.

[2]Percent calories from fat = (total fat calories divided by total calories) multiplied by 100; total fat calories = total fat (grams) multiplied by 9.

oz. = ounce

Product (3½ Ounces, Cooked)*	Saturated Fatty Acids (Grams)	Cholesterol (Milligrams)	Fat[1] (Grams)	Calories From Fat[2] (%)	Total Calories
Feta, 1 oz.	4.2	25	6.0	72	75
Neufchatel, 1 oz.	4.2	22	6.6	81	74
Camembert, 1 oz.	4.3	20	6.9	73	85
American processed cheese food, pasteurized, 1 oz.	4.4	18	7.0	68	93
Provolone, 1 oz.	4.8	20	7.6	68	100
Limburger, 1 oz.	4.8	26	7.7	75	93
Brie, 1 oz.	4.9	28	7.9	74	95
Romano, 1 oz.	4.9	29	7.6	63	110
Gouda, 1 oz.	5.0	32	7.8	69	101
Swiss, 1 oz.	5.0	26	7.8	65	107
Edam, 1 oz.	5.0	25	7.9	70	101
Brick, 1 oz.	5.3	27	8.4	72	105
Blue, 1 oz.	5.3	21	8.2	73	100
Gruyere, 1 oz.	5.4	31	9.2	71	117
Muenster, 1 oz.	5.4	27	8.5	74	104
Parmesan, 1 oz.	5.4	22	8.5	59	129
Monterey Jack, 1 oz.	5.5	25	8.6	73	106
Roquefort, 1 oz.	5.5	26	8.7	75	105
Ricotta, part-skim, 4 oz.	5.6	25	9.0	52	156
American processed cheese, pasteurized, 1 oz.	5.6	27	8.9	75	106
Colby, 1 oz.	5.7	27	9.1	73	112
Cheddar, 1 oz.	6.0	30	9.4	74	114
Cream cheese, 1 oz.	6.2	31	9.9	90	99
Ricotta, whole milk, 4 oz.	9.4	58	14.7	67	197
Eggs					
Egg, chicken, white	0	0	tr.	0	16
Egg, chicken, whole	1.7	274	5.6	64	79
Egg, chicken, yolk	1.7	272	5.6	80	63

tr. = trace

Source:
Composition of Foods: Dairy and Egg Products - Raw • Processed • Prepared, Agriculture Handbook 8-1, United States Department of Agriculture, Agricultural Research Service (November 1976).

FATS AND OILS

Fats and oils are a major source of saturated fat in the diet. With the exceptions of lard, butter, and beef tallow, fats and oils are not sources of cholesterol. You will want to choose products with the highest polyunsaturated and lowest saturated fat content. This table lists the saturated fat, cholesterol, polyunsaturated fat, and monounsaturated fat content of selected fats and oils.

Product (1 tablespoon)	Saturated Fatty Acids (Grams)	Cholesterol (Milligrams)	Poly-unsaturated Fatty Acids (Grams)	Mono-unsaturated Fatty Acids (Grams)
Rapeseed oil (canola oil)	0.9	0	4.5	7.6
Safflower oil	1.2	0	10.1	1.6
Sunflower oil	1.4	0	5.5	6.2
Peanut butter, smooth	1.5	0	2.3	3.7
Corn oil	1.7	0	8.0	3.3
Olive oil	1.8	0	1.1	9.9
Hydrogenated sunflower oil	1.8	0	4.9	6.3
Margarine, liquid, bottled	1.8	0	5.1	3.9
Margarine, soft, tub	1.8	0	3.9	4.8
Sesame oil	1.9	0	5.7	5.4
Soybean oil	2.0	0	7.9	3.2
Margarine, stick	2.1	0	3.6	5.1
Peanut oil	2.3	0	4.3	6.2
Cottonseed oil	3.5	0	7.1	2.4
Lard	5.0	12	1.4	5.8
Beef tallow	6.4	14	0.5	5.3
Palm oil	6.7	0	1.3	5.0
Butter	7.1	31	0.4	3.3
Cocoa butter	8.1	0	0.4	4.5
Palm kernel oil	11.1	0	0.2	1.5
Coconut oil	11.8	0	0.2	0.8

BREADS, CEREALS, PASTA, RICE, DRIED PEAS, AND BEANS

The following table gives the saturated fat, cholesterol, total fat, calories from fat, and total calorie content of selected breads, cereals, pasta, rice, dried peas and beans. Select those items that are low in saturated fat and cholesterol.

Product	Saturated Fatty Acids (Grams)	Cholesterol (Milligrams)	Total Fat[1] (Grams)	Calories From Fat[2] (%)	Total Calories
Breads					
Melba toast, 1 plain	0.1	0	tr.	0	20
Pita, 1/2 large shell	0.1	0	1.0	5	165
Corn tortilla	0.1	0	1.0	14	65
Rye bread, 1 slice	0.2	0	1.0	14	65
English muffin	0.3	0	1.0	6	140
Bagel, 1, 3 1/2"diamater	0.3	0	1.0	6	140
White bread, 1 slice	0.3	0	1.0	14	65
Rye krisp, 2 triple crackers	0.3	0	1.0	16	56
Whole wheat bread, 1 slice	0.4	0	1.0	13	70
Saltines, 4	0.5	4	1.0	18	50
Hamburger bun	0.5	tr.	2.0	16	115
Hot dog bun	0.5	tr.	2.0	16	115
Pancake, 1, 4" diameter	0.5	16	2.0	30	60
Bran muffin, 1, 2 1/2" diameter	1.4	24	6.0	43	125

[1]Total fat = saturated fatty acids plus monounsaturated fatty acids plus polyunsaturated fatty acids.

[2]Percent calories from fat = (total fat calories divided by total calories) multiplied by 100; total fat calories = total fat (grams) multiplied by 9.

oz. = ounce

tr. = trace

Product	Saturated Fatty Acids (Grams)	Cholesterol (Milligrams)	Total Fat[1] (Grams)	Calories From Fat[2] (%)	Total Calories
Corn muffin, 1, 2¹/₂" diameter	1.5	23	5.0	31	145
Plain doughnut, 1, 3¹/₄" diameter	2.8	20	12.0	51	210
Croissant, 1, 4¹/₂" by 4"	3.5	13	12.0	46	235
Waffle, 1, 7" diameter	4.0	102	13.0	48	245
Cereals (1 cup)					
Corn flakes	tr.	—	0.1	0	98
Cream of wheat, cooked	tr.	—	0.5	3	134
Corn grits, cooked	tr.	—	0.5	3	146
Oatmeal, cooked	0.4	—	2.4	15	145
Granola	5.8	—	33.1	50	595
100% Natural Cereal with raisins and dates	13.7	—	20.3	37	496
Pasta (1 cup)					
Spaghetti, cooked	0.1	0	1.0	6	155
Elbow macaroni, cooked	0.1	0	1.0	6	155
Egg noodles, cooked	0.5	50	2.0	11	160
Chow mein noodles, canned	2.1	5	11.0	45	220
Rice (1 cup cooked)					
Rice, white	0.1	0	0.5	2	225
Rice, brown	0.3	0	1.0	4	230
Dried Peas and Beans (1 cup cooked)					
Split peas	0.1	0	0.8	3	231
Kidney beans	0.1	0	1.0	4	225
Lima beans	0.2	0	0.7	3	217
Black eyed peas	0.3	0	1.2	5	200
Garbanzo beans	0.4	0	4.3	14	269

— = Information not available in sources used.

Sources:

Composition of Foods: Breakfast Cereals - Raw • Processed • Prepared. Agriculture Handbook 8-16. United States Department of Agriculture, Nutrition Monitoring Division (December 1986).

Home and Garden Bulletin. Nutritive Value of Foods. No. 72. United States Department of Agriculture. Human Nutrition Information Service (1986).

SWEETS, SNACKS, AND FROZEN DESSERTS

The total dietary plan for lowering cholesterol includes limiting cholesterol, saturated fats, and weight control. To help you take control of cholesterol, the table table below lists the saturated fat, cholesterol, total fat, calories from fat, and total calorie content of common sweets, snacks, and frozen desserts.

Product	Saturated Fatty Acids (Grams)	Cholesterol (Milligrams)	Total Fat[1] (Grams)	Calories From Fat[2] (%)	Total Calories
Beverages					
Ginger ale, 12 oz.	0.0	0	0.0	0	125
Cola, regular, 12 oz.	0.0	0	0.0	0	160
Chocolate shake, 10 oz.	6.5	37	10.5	26	360
Candy (1 ounce)					
Hard candy	0.0	0	0.0	0	110
Gum drops	tr.	0	tr.	tr.	100
Fudge	2.1	1	3.0	24	115
Milk chocolate, plain	5.4	6	9.0	56	145
Cookies					
Vanilla wafers, 5 cookies, 1³/₄" diameter	0.9	12	3.3	32	94
Fig bars, 4 cookies 1⁵/₈" × 1⁵/₈" × ³/₈"	1.0	27	4.0	17	210
Chocolate brownie with icing, 1¹/₂" by 1³/₄" by ⁷/₈"	1.6	14	4.0	36	100

[1]Total fat = saturated fatty acids plus monounsaturated fatty acids plus polyunsaturated fatty acids.

[2]Percent calories from fat = (total fat calories divided by total calories) multiplied by 100; total fat calories = total fat (grams) multiplied by 9.

— = Information not available in sources used.

oz. = ounce

tr. = trace

Product	Saturated Fatty Acids (Grams)	Cholesterol (Milligrams)	Total Fat[1] (Grams)	Calories From Fat[2] (%)	Total Calories
Oatmeal cookies, 4 cookies, 2⅝" diameter	2.5	2	10.0	37	245
Chocolate chip cookies, 4 cookies, 2¼" diameter	3.9	18	11.0	54	185
Cakes and Pies					
Angel food cake, 1/12 of 10" cake	tr.	0	tr.	125	125
Gingerbread, 1/9 of 8" cake	1.1	1	4.0	21	175
White layer cake with white icing, 1/16 of 9" cake	2.1	3	9.0	32	260
Yellow layer cake with chocolate icing, 1/16 of 9" cake	3.0	36	8.0	31	235
Pound cake, 1/17 of loaf	3.0	64	5.0	41	110
Devils food cake with chocolate icing, 1/16 of 9" cake	3.5	37	8.0	31	235
Lemon meringue pie, 1/6 of 9" pie	4.3	143	14.0	36	355
Apple pie, 1/6 of 9" pie	4.6	0	18.0	40	405
Cream pie, 1/6 of 9" pie	15.0	8	23.0	46	455
Snacks					
Popcorn, air-popped, 1 cup	tr.	0	tr.	tr.	30
Pretzels, stick, 2¼", 10 pretzels	tr.	0	tr.	tr.	10
Popcorn with oil and salted, 1 cup	0.5	0	3.0	49	55
Corn chips, 1 oz.	1.4	25	9.0	52	155
Potato chips, 1 oz.	2.6	0	10.1	62	147
Pudding					
Gelatin	0.0	0	0.0	0	70

Product	Saturated Fatty Acids (Grams)	Cholesterol (Milligrams)	Total Fat[1] (Grams)	Calories From Fat[2] (%)	Total Calories
Tapioca, $^1/_2$ cup	2.3	15	4.0	25	145
Chocolate pudding, $^1/_2$ cup	2.4	15	4.0	24	150
Fruit popsicle, 1 bar	—	—	0.0	0	65
Fruit ice	—	—	tr.	0	247
Fudgsicle	—	—	0.2	2	91
Frozen yogurt, fruit flavored	—	—	2.0	8	216
Sherbet, orange	2.4	14	3.8	13	270
Pudding pops, 1 pop	2.5	1	2.6	25	94
Ice milk, vanilla, soft serve	2.9	13	4.6	19	223
Ice milk, vanilla, hard	3.5	18	5.6	28	184
Ice cream, vanilla, regular	8.9	59	14.3	48	269
Ice cream, french vanilla, soft serve	13.5	153	22.5	54	377
Ice cream, vanilla, rich, 16% fat	14.7	88	23.7	61	349

Sources:

Composition of Foods: Dairy and Egg Products - Raw • Processed • Prepared, Agriculture Handbook 8-1. United States Department of Agriculture, Agricultural Research Service (November 1976).

Pennington, J., and Church, H. *Bowes and Church's Food Values of Portions Commonly Used.* 14th ed. Philadelphia: J.B. Lippincott Company (1985).

Home and Garden Bulletin. Nutritive Value of Foods. United States Department of Agriculture. Human Nutrition Information Service (1986).

NUTS AND SEEDS

Choose those nuts and seeds that are lowest in saturated fats when following a low cholesterol, low-fat diet plan. This table gives you the saturated fat, cholesterol, total fat, calories from fat, and total calorie content of some nut and seed products.

Product (1 ounce)	Saturated Fatty Acids (Grams)	Cholesterol (Milligrams)	Total Fat[1] (Grams)	Calories From Fat[2] (%)	Total Calories
European chestnuts	0.2	0	1.1	9	105
Filberts or Hazelnuts	1.3	0	17.8	89	179
Almonds	1.4	0	15.0	80	167
Pecans	1.5	0	18.4	89	187
Sunflower seed kernels, roasted	1.5	0	1.4	77	165
English walnuts	1.6	0	17.6	87	182
Pistachio nuts	1.7	0	13.7	75	164
Peanuts	1.9	0	14.0	76	164
Hickory nuts	2.0	0	18.3	88	187
Pine nuts, pignolia	2.2	0	14.4	89	146
Pumpkin and squash seed kernels	2.3	0	12.0	73	148
Cashew nuts	2.8	0	13.2	73	163
Macadamia nuts	3.1	0	20.9	95	199
Brazil nuts	4.6	0	18.8	91	186
Coconut meat, unsweetened	16.3	0	18.3	88	187

[1]Total fat = saturated fatty acids plus monounsaturated fatty acids plus polyunsaturated fatty acids.

[2]Percent calories from fat = (total fat calories divided by total calories) multiplied by 100; total fat calories = total fat (grams) multiplied by 9.

Composition of Foods: Legumes and Legume Products Raw • Processed • Prepared, Agriculture Handbook 8-16. United States Department of Agriculture, Human Nutrition Information Service (December 1986).

Composition of Foods: Nut and Seed Products - Raw • Processed • Prepared, Agriculture Handbook 8-12. United States Department of Agriculture, Human Nutrition Information Service (September 1984).

MISCELLANEOUS ITEMS

The following table provides the saturated fat, cholesterol, total fat, calories from fat, and total calorie content of miscellaneous food items. This information may be benefi-

cial to you, in adhering to a low cholesterol, low fat saturated fat diet.

Product	Saturated Fatty Acids (Grams)	Cholesterol (Milligrams)	Total Fat[1] (Grams)	Calories From Fat[2] (%)	Total Calories
Gravies (1/2 cup)					
Au jus, canned	0.1	1	0.3	3	80
Turkey, canned	0.7	3	2.5	37	61
Beef, canned	1.4	4	2.8	41	62
Chicken, canned	1.7	3	6.8	65	95
Sauces (1/2 cup)					
Sweet and sour	tr.	0	0.1	? 1	147
Barbecue	0.3	0	2.3	22	94
White	3.2	17	6.7	50	121
Cheese	4.7	26	8.6	50	154
Sour cream	8.5	45	15.1	53	255
Hollandaise	20.9	94	34.1	87	353
Bearnaise	20.9	99	34.1	88	351
Salad Dressings (1 Tablespoon)					
Russian, low calorie	0.1	1	0.7	27	23
French, low calorie	0.1	1	0.9	37	22
Italian, low calorie	0.2	1	1.5	85	16
Thousand Island, low calorie	0.2	2	1.6	59	24
Imitation mayonnaise	0.5	4	2.9	75	35
Thousand Island, regular	0.9	—	5.6	86	59
Italian, regular	1.0	—	7.1	93	69

[1]Total fat = saturated fatty acids plus monounsaturated fatty acids plus polyunsaturated fatty acids.

[2]Percent calories from fat = (total fat calories divided by total calories) multiplied by 100; total fat calories = total fat (grams) multiplied by 9.

— = Information not available in the sources used.

Product	Saturated Fatty Acids (Grams)	Cholesterol Milligrams	Total Fat[1] (Grams)	Calories From Fat[2] (%)	Total Calories
Russian, regular	1.1	—	7.8	92	76
French, regular	1.5	—	6.4	86	67
Blue cheese	1.5	—	8.0	93	77
Mayonnaise	1.6	8	11.0	100	99
Other					
Olives, green 4 medium	0.2	0	1.5	90	15
Nondairy creamer powdered, 1 teaspoon	0.7	0	1.0	90	10
Liquid, 1/2 oz.	less than 1 gm.	0	2.0	12.2	20
Avocado, Florida	5.3	0	27.0	72	340
Pizza, cheese, 1/8 of 15" diameter	4.1	56	9.0	28	290
Quiche lorraine, 1/8 of 8" diameter	23.2	285	48.0	72	600

Sources:

Composition of Foods: Fats and Oils - Raw • Processed • Prepared, Agriculture Handbook 8-4. United States Department of Agriculture, Science and Education Administration (June 1979).

Composition of Foods: Soups, Sauces and Gravies - Raw • Processed • Prepared, Agriculture Handbook 8-6. United States Department of Agriculture, Science and Education Administration (February 1980).

Home and Garden Bulletin. Nutritive Value of Foods. No. 72. United States Department of Agriculture. Human Nutrition Information Service (1986).

Appendix 3

Flow Charts

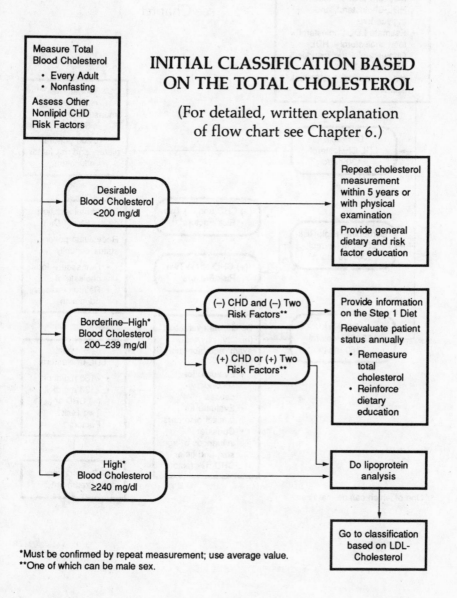

INITIAL CLASSIFICATION BASED ON THE TOTAL CHOLESTEROL

(For detailed, written explanation of flow chart see Chapter 6.)

Measure Total Blood Cholesterol
- Every Adult
- Nonfasting

Assess Other Nonlipid CHD Risk Factors

Desirable Blood Cholesterol <200 mg/dl

Repeat cholesterol measurement within 5 years or with physical examination

Provide general dietary and risk factor education

Borderline–High* Blood Cholesterol 200–239 mg/dl

(–) CHD and (–) Two Risk Factors**

(+) CHD or (+) Two Risk Factors**

Provide information on the Step 1 Diet

Reevaluate patient status annually
- Remeasure total cholesterol
- Reinforce dietary education

High* Blood Cholesterol ≥240 mg/dl

Do lipoprotein analysis

Go to classification based on LDL-Cholesterol

*Must be confirmed by repeat measurement; use average value.
**One of which can be male sex.

CLASSIFICATION BASED ON LDL CHOLESTEROL

(For detailed, written explanation of flow chart see Chapter 6.)

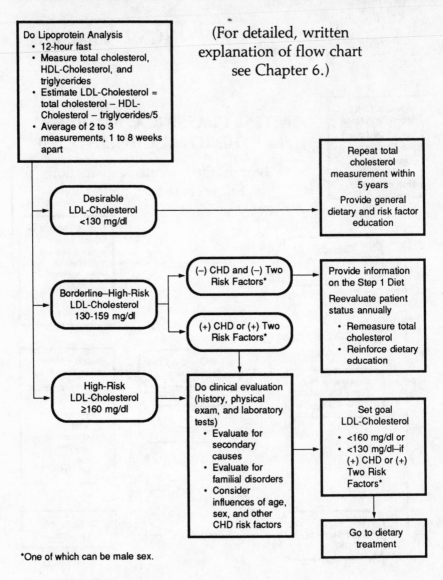

Do Lipoprotein Analysis
- 12-hour fast
- Measure total cholesterol, HDL-Cholesterol, and triglycerides
- Estimate LDL-Cholesterol = total cholesterol − HDL-Cholesterol − triglycerides/5
- Average of 2 to 3 measurements, 1 to 8 weeks apart

Desirable LDL-Cholesterol <130 mg/dl

Repeat total cholesterol measurement within 5 years

Provide general dietary and risk factor education

Borderline–High-Risk LDL-Cholesterol 130-159 mg/dl

(−) CHD and (−) Two Risk Factors*

(+) CHD or (+) Two Risk Factors*

Provide information on the Step 1 Diet

Reevaluate patient status annually
- Remeasure total cholesterol
- Reinforce dietary education

High-Risk LDL-Cholesterol ≥160 mg/dl

Do clinical evaluation (history, physical exam, and laboratory tests)
- Evaluate for secondary causes
- Evaluate for familial disorders
- Consider influences of age, sex, and other CHD risk factors

Set goal LDL-Cholesterol
- <160 mg/dl or
- <130 mg/dl–if (+) CHD or (+) Two Risk Factors*

Go to dietary treatment

*One of which can be male sex.

DIETARY TREATMENT PLAN

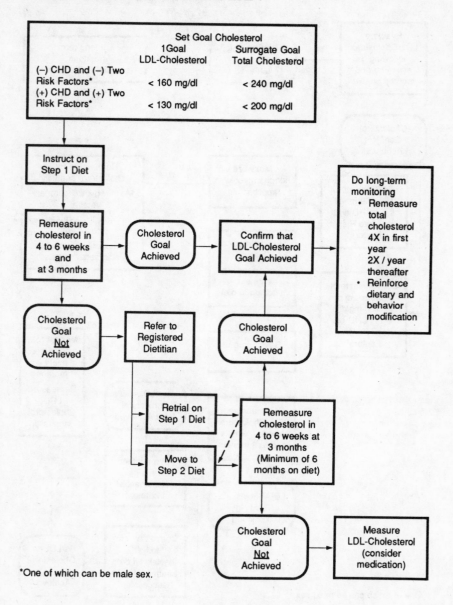

*One of which can be male sex.

MEDICATION TREATMENT PLAN

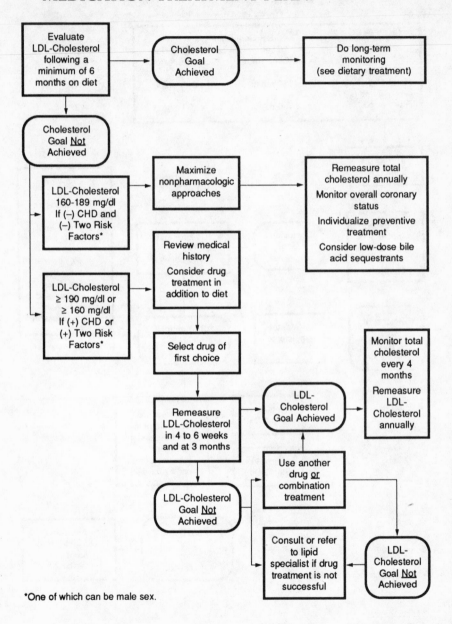

*One of which can be male sex.

Appendix 4

Metropolitan Life Height and Weight Table

Desirable weights for adults age 25 and older*
(weights listed in tables in pounds without clothing).

Height without shoes (Feet)	(Inches)	Small	Frame Medium	Large
Men				
5	1	123–129	126–136	133–145
5	2	125–131	128–138	135–148
5	3	127–133	130–140	137–151
5	4	129–135	132–143	139–155
5	5	131–137	134–146	141–159
5	6	133–140	137–149	144–163
5	7	135–143	140–152	147–167
5	8	137–146	143–155	150–171
5	9	139–149	146–158	153–175
5	10	141–152	149–161	157–179
5	11	144–155	152–165	159–183
6	0	147–159	155–169	163–187
6	1	150–163	159–173	167–192
6	2	153–167	162–177	171–197
6	3	157–171	166–182	176–202

*For persons 18–24 years subtract 1 pound for each year under 25 years of age.

| Height without shoes | | | Frame | |
(Feet)	(Inches)	Small	Medium	Large
Women				
4	9	99–108	106–118	115–128
4	10	100–110	108–120	117–131
4	11	101–112	110–123	119–134
5	0	103–115	112–126	122–137
5	1	105–118	115–129	125–140
5	2	108–121	118–132	128–144
5	3	111–124	121–135	131–148
5	4	114–127	124–138	134–152
5	5	117–130	127–141	137–156
5	6	120–133	130–144	140–160
5	7	123–136	133–147	143-164
5	8	126–139	136–150	146–167
5	9	129–142	139–153	149–170
5	10	132-145	142–156	152–173
5	11	135–148	145–159	155–176

Courtesy of The Metropolitan Life Insurance Company, New York, New York. Weight charts based on 1983 actuarial tables.

Appendix 5

Fast Food Tables

The following tables provide information about the calorie content, total fat and saturated fat content of selected fast foods. In Table One, the food items are arranged in restaurant groups. If you frequently eat at a particular fast food restaurant and would like to know about their menu items, they will be easy to find in Table One. In Table Two of the fast food information section, foods are listed according to menu items. If you are interested in eating a roast beef sandwich and want to see how various restaurants compare, you will find Table Two, provides the best and easiest information.

The last portion of the fast food information section lists the addresses of several fast food chains. If you would like a complete listing of that restaurant's menu items, you can write to the address listed, or inquire at your local restaurant. Much of the calorie and fat content information for fast food restaurants, change due to different suppliers, varied cooking techniques, and substituting products. If you have any questions, ask at the local restaurant or write to the addresses listed on page 159.

Food Product	Weight	Calories	Total Fat Grams	Saturated Fat	Fat Calories
Arby's (regular roast beef)	5 oz.	365	19	7 grams	47%
Arby's Chicken Breast Sandwich	7 oz.	567	32	7 Grams	51%
Arby's French Fries	3 oz.	222	11	3 Grams	45%
Arby's Chocolate Shake	11 oz.	426	14	7 Grams	30%
Burger King Whopper	9 oz.	584	33	13 Grams	51%
Burger King Whaler	6 oz.	478	26	3 Grams	49%
Burger King Chicken Tenders	3 oz.	223	12	3 Grams	48%
Burger King French Fries	3 oz.	255	13	5 Grams	46%
Burger King Chocolate Shake	11 oz.	351	10	5 Grams	26%
Church's Fried Chicken (2 piece)	6 oz.	487	35	9 Grams	65%
Church's Fried Chicken Fries	4 oz.	338	16	5 Grams	43%
Hardee's Roast Beef (regular)	5 oz.	338	17	6 Grams	45%
Hardee's Chicken Filet Sandwich	7 oz.	431	20	6 Grams	42%
Hardee's French Fries	3 oz.	230	12	4 Grams	47%
Hardee's Chocolate Shake	11 oz.	349	11	6 Grams	28%
McDonald's Big Mac	7 oz.	572	34	15 Grams	53%
McDonald's Filet-O-Fish	4 oz.	415	23	5 Grams	50%
McDonald's Chicken McNuggets	4 oz.	283	18	5 Grams	57%
McDonald's French Fries	3 oz.	222	12	5 Grams	49%
McDonald's Chocolate Shake	11 oz.	356	10	6 Grams	25%
Kentucky Fried Chicken (2 piece)	6 oz.	460	31	7 Grams	61%
Kentucky Fried Chicken Nuggets	4 oz.	281	17	4 Grams	54%

Food Product	Weight	Calories	Total Fat Grams	Saturated Fat	Fat Calories
Kentucky Fried Chicken French Fries	3 oz.	249	13	2 Grams	47%
Roy Roger's Roast Beef	6 oz.	335	11	3 Grams	30%
Roy Roger's Chicken (2 piece)	6 oz.	519	35	8 Grams	61%
Roy Roger's French Fries	3 oz.	237	13	4 Grams	49%
Roy Roger's Chocolate Shake	12 oz.	430	11	6 Grams	23%
Wendy's Big Classic	8 oz.	500	28	11 Grams	50%
Wendy's Chicken Filet Sandwich	8 oz.	479	24	7 Grams	45%
Wendy's French Fries	3 oz.	287	14	4 Grams	44%
Wendy's Chocolate Frosty	9 oz.	351	13	6 Grams	33%

Menu Item	Weight	Calories	Total Fat Grams	Saturated Fat Grams	Fat Calories
Hamburgers					
Burger King Whopper	9 oz.	584	33	13	51%
McDonald's Big Mac	7 oz.	572	34	15	53%
Wendy's Big Classic	8 oz.	500	28	11	50%
Roast Beef					
Arby's (regular)	5 oz.	365	19	7	47%
Hardee's (regular)	5 oz.	338	17	6	45%
Roy Roger's	6 oz.	335	11	3	30%
Fish					
Burger King Whaler	6 oz.	478	26	3	49%
McDonald's Filet-O-Fish	5 oz.	415	23	5	50%
Chicken					
Arby's Chicken Breast Sandwich	7 oz.	567	32	7	51%
Burger King Chicken Tenders	3 oz.	223	12	3	48%

Menu Item	Weight	Calories	Total Fat Grams	Saturated Fat Grams	Fat Calories
Church's Fried Chicken 2 piece	6 oz.	487	35	9	65%
Hardee's Chicken Filet Sandwich	7 oz.	431	20	6	42%
Kentucky Fried Chicken 2 piece	6 oz.	460	31	7	61%
Kentucky Fried Chicken Nuggets	4 oz.	281	18	5	58%
Roy Roger's Chicken 2 piece	6 oz.	519	35	8	61%
Wendy's Chicken Sandwich	8 oz.	479	24	7	45%
French Fries					
Arby's	3 oz.	222	11	3	45%
Burger King	3 oz.	255	13	5	46%
Church's Fried Chicken	4 oz.	338	16	5	43%
Hardee's	3 oz.	230	12	4	47%
Kentucky Fried Chicken	3 oz.	249	13	2	47%
McDonald's	3 oz.	222	12	5	49%
Roy Rogers	3 oz.	237	13	4	49%
Wendy's	3 oz.	287	14	4	44%
Chocolate Shakes					
Arby's	11 oz.	426	14	7	30%
Burger King	11 oz.	351	10	5	26%
Hardee's	11 oz.	349	11	6	28%
McDonald's	11 oz.	356	10	6	25%
Roy Rogers	12 oz.	430	11	6	23%
Wendy's Frosty	9 oz.	351	13	6	33%

Fast Food Addresses

Arby's
Consumer Affairs,
Arby's Inc.
Ten Piedmont Center, Suite 700
3495 Piedmont Road
Atlanta, Georgia 30305

Burger King
Consumer Information,
Burger King Corporation
1777 Old Cutler Road
Miami, Florida 33157

**Frisch's Big Boy Restaurant
Incorporated**
Consumer Affairs Office
2800 Gilbert Avenue
Cincinnati, Ohio 45206

Hardee's
Hardee Food Systems
P.O. Box 1619
Rocky Mount, North Carolina
27804-2805

Kentucky Fried Chicken
Public Affairs Department
KFC Corporation
P.O. Box 32070
Louisville, Kentucky 40232

McDonald's
McDonald's Nutrition
Information Center
McDonald's Plaza
Oak Brook, Illinois 60521

Pizza Hut
Pizza Hut
Information Center
P.O. Box 484
911 East Douglas
Wichita, Kansas 67202

RAX
RAX Restaurants
Consumer Affairs
1317 East Broad Street
Columbus, Ohio 43205

Roy Rogers
Roy Rogers Division of
Frisch's Big Boy Restaurants
Consumer Affairs Office
2800 Gilbert Avenue
Cincinnati, Ohio 45206

Wendy's
Consumer Affairs
Department
Wendy's International, Inc.
P.O. Box 256
Dublin, Ohio 43017

For questions or additional information please write to us at:

Heartsmart
P.O. Box 42346
Cincinnati, Ohio 45242

Be sure to include your question along with your name and address and we will answer questions or provide additional information to you.

Selected References

Chapter 1

American Heart Association. *Heart Facts 1987*

Lipid Research Clinics Program: The Lipid Research Clinics Coronary Primary Prevention Trial results: I. Reduction in the incidence of coronary heart disease. JAMA 1984;251:351-364

Lipid Research Clinics Program: The Lipid Research Clinics Coronary Primary Prevention Trial results: II. The relationship of reduction in incidence of coronary heart disease to cholesterol lowering. JAMA 1984;251:365-374

National Institutes of Health Consensus Development Conference Statement Vol. 5; No. 7: Lowering Blood Cholesterol to Prevent Heart Disease. 1984; U.S. Department of Health and Human Services, National Institutes of Health Office of Medical Applications of Research, Building 1, Room 216, Bethesda, Maryland 20205

Stamler J, Wentworth D, Neaton J, et al: Is Relationship Between Serum Cholesterol and Risk of Premature Death from Coronary Heart Disease Continuous or Graded? JAMA 1986;256:2823-2828

Chapter 2

American Academy of Pediatrics Committee on Nutrition: Prudent Life-style for Children: Dietary Fat and Cholesterol. Pediatrics 1986;78:521-525

Grundy S: Cholesterol and Coronary Heart Disease A New Era. JAMA 1986;256:2849-2858

Report of the National Cholesterol Education Program Expert Panel on Detection, Evaluation, and Treatment of High Blood Cholesterol in Adults. Archives Internal Medicine 1988;148: 36-69

Rudel L, Parks J, Johnson F, Babiak J: Low Density Lipoproteins in Atherosclerosis. Journal of Lipid Research 1986;27:465-474

Thuesen L, Henriksen L, Engby B: One-year Experience with a Low-fat, Low-cholesterol Diet in Patients with Coronary Heart Disease. The American Journal of Clinical Nutrition 1986; 44:212-219

U.S. Department of Health and Human Services, Public Health Service, National Institutes of Health. Cholesterol Counts: Steps to Lowering Your Patient's Blood Cholesterol; Cholesterol Management Principles from the Coronary Primary Prevention Trial. NIH Publication No. 85-2699

Wynder E, Field F, Haley N: Population Screening for Cholesterol Determination: A Pilot Study. JAMA 1986; 256: 2839-2842

Chapter 3

Ballard-Barbash R, Callaway C.W: Marine Fish Oils: Role in Prevention of Coronary Artery Disease. Mayo Clinic Proceedings 1987; 62:113-118

Becker D, Brown Wilder L, Pearson T: Hypercholesterolemia: Nutritional and Pharmacologic Management. Maryland Medical Association Journal 1986; 35:549-551

Grundy S: Comparison of Monounsaturated Fatty Acids and Carbohydrates for Plasma Cholesterol Lowering. New England Journal of Medicine 1986; 314: 745-748

Keys A: Serum Cholesterol Response to Dietary Cholesterol. American Journal of Clinical Nutrition 1984;40:351-359

Kinsella J: Dietary Fish Oils. Nutrition Today 1986; Nov.-Dec.:7-14

Mattson F, Grundy S: Comparison of Dietary Saturated, Monounsaturated, and Polyunsaturated Fatty Acids on Plasma Lipids and Lipoproteins in Man. Journal Lipid Research 1985; 26:194-202

Nutrition and the M.D. A Continuing Education Service for Physicians and Nutritionists. 1986;12

U.S. Department of Health and Human Services, Public Health Service, National Institutes of Health. *Facts About Blood Cholesterol.* NIH Publication No. 85-2696

Chapter 4

American Heart Association. *An Eating Plan for Healthy Americans.* AHA publication 51-018-B(SA)

American Heart Association. Dietary Guidelines for Healthy American Adults: A Statement for Physicians and Health Professionals by the Nutrition Committee, American Heart Association. Circulation 1986;74:1465A-1468A

American Heart Association. *Eating for a Healthy Heart.* Dietary Treatment of Hyperlipidemia. AHA publication 50-063-A

American Heart Association. *The Way to a Man's Heart.* AHA publication 51-08-A

Consensus Development Conference: Lowering Blood Cholesterol to Prevent Heart Disease. JAMA 1985;253:2080-2086

Grundy S, Bilheimer D, Blackburn H, et al: Rationale of the Diet Heart Statement of the American Heart Association: Report of Nutrition Committee. Circulation 1982;65:839A-854A

U.S. Department of Health and Human Services, Public Health Service, National Institutes of Health: So you have high blood cholesterol . . . ; NIH publication No. 87-2922

Chapter 6

Report of the National Cholesterol Education Program Expert Panel on Detection, Evaluation, and Treatment of High Blood Cholesterol in Adults. Archives of Internal Medicine 1988; 148:36-69

U.S. Department of Health and Human Services, Public Health Service, National Institutes of Health publication No. 87-2920

U.S. Department of Health and Human Services, Public Health Service, National Institutes of Health. Cholesterol Management Principles from the Coronary Primary Prevention Trial; NIH publication No. 85-2699

Lowering Blood Cholesterol to Prevent Heart Disease. National Institutes of Health Consensus Development Conference Statement; Vol. 5, No. 7

Chapter 7

Glueck C: Drugs that Affect High-Density Lipoprotein Cholesterol Levels: Mechanisms of Action and Relationships to Coronary Heart Disease. Internal Medicine 1985 special issue; 20-25

Report of the National Cholesterol Education Program Expert Panel on Detection, Evaluation, and Treatment of High Blood Cholesterol in Adults. Archives of Internal Medicine 1988; 148:36-69

Chapter 8

Anderson K, Castelli W, Levy D: Cholesterol and Mortality: 30 Years of Follow-up from the Framingham Study. JAMA 1987. 257: 2176-2180

Castelli W: Cardiovascular Disease and Multifactorial Risk: Challenge of the 1980s. American Heart Journal 1983. 106:1191-1200

Dwyer J, et al. Low Level Cigarette Smoking and Logitudinal Change in Serum Cholesterol Among Adolescents, The Berlin-Bremen Study. JAMA 1988;259:2857-2862

Multiple Risk Factor Intervention Trial Research Group: Coronary Heart Disease, Death, Nonfatal Acute Myocardial Infarction and Other Clinical Outcomes in the Multiple Risk Factor Intervention Trial: American Journal of Cardiology 1986; 58:1-9

Multiple Risk Factor Intervention Trial Research Group: Multiple Risk Factor Intervention Trial, Risk Factor Changes and Mortality Results: JAMA 1982;248:1465-1477

Chapter 9

Coronary Drug Project Research Group: Colfibrate and niacin in coronary heart disease. JAMA 1975;231:360-381

Helsinki Heart Study: Primary Prevention Trial with Gemfibrozil in Middle-aged Men with Dyslipidemia. New England Journal of Medicine 1987;317:

Lipid Research Clinics Coronary Primary Prevention Trial Results: I. Reduction in incidence of coronary disease. II. The relationship of reduction in incidence of coronary heart disease to cholesterol lowering. JAMA 1984 251:351-365

Lovastatin Study Group: Therapeutic response to lovastatin (mevinolin) in nonfamilial hypercholesterolemia. JAMA 1986; 256:2829-2834

Shepherd J, et al: Effects of nicotinic acid therapy on plasma high-density lipoprotein subfraction distribution and composition and on appoliprotein A metabolism. Journal of Clinical Investigation 1979;63:858-862

Shepherd J, et al: The effects of cholestyramine on high-density lipoprotein metabolism. Atherosclerosis 1979;33:433

Vega G, Grundy S: Treatment of primary moderate hypercholesterolemia with lovastatin (mevinolin) and Colestipol. JAMA 1987;257:33-38

Chapter 10

American Heart Association: "Dining Out: a guide to restaurant dining." AHA publication 50-067(CP)

Chapter 11

Diet for a Healthy Heart: Fleischmann's for Nabisco Brands, Inc. 1985

American Heart Association: Recipes for fat-controlled, low-cholesterol meals. AHA publication 50-020(CP)

The American Heart Association Cookbook, 4th ed, M Winston, R. Eshleman, 1984. David McKay Co., New York

Glossary

Angina Pectoris   A reversible condition in which the heart muscle temporarily does not receive a sufficient supply of blood. This decreased blood supply to the heart occurs when the coronary arteries are blocked with cholesterol and fatty deposits, limiting the supply that is necessary for the heart to function. When restricted blood flow to the heart occurs, the person may experience discomfort, most typically in the chest. This discomfort may be in the chest, arm, shoulder, back, or neck and may be described as pressure, burning, aching, or a squeezing pain.

Atherosclerosis   This condition is commonly called "hardening of the arteries." It is a progressive disease that causes the arteries to become narrowed and the walls of the arteries to lose their elasticity. The arteries are narrowed and hardened when cholesterol and fats build up in the walls of the arteries. When atherosclerosis occurs in the coronary arteries, the heart muscle does not receive the blood and nutrients it needs, and this leads to angina pectoris, and possibly heart attack.

Bile Acid Sequestrants   One of the first line medications that may be used to treat an abnormally high cholesterol level. The bile acid sequestrants bind the cholesterol contained in the bile acids in the intestine. When the cholesterol has been bound by the bile acid sequestrant, it is eliminated from the body in the stool.

167

Cholesterol A fatty substance that is necessary for many body functions. It is manufactured by the human body and by all animals as well as fish and fowl.

Blood Cholesterol All cholesterol that is found in the blood. Blood cholesterol is the cholesterol that the body manufactures in addition to the cholesterol you eat. The cholesterol in the blood is one factor in the development of atherosclerosis.

Dietary Cholesterol Cholesterol that is found in the foods you eat. Dietary cholesterol is found only in foods from animal sources. Dietary cholesterol contributes to the elevation of blood cholesterol and the subsequent development of atherosclerosis.

Coronary Arteries The blood vessels that carry blood rich in oxygen and nutrients to the heart. When the coronary arteries become narrowed with atherosclerosis, angina pectoris and heart attack can occur. Any disease of the coronary arteries is referred to as coronary artery disease.

Diabetes A chronic disease that affects the body's use of carbohydrates and fats. People with diabetes often have abnormal blood cholesterol values.

Diuretic A medication that is used to increase the production of urine. Frequently referred to as a water pill, diuretics may be used to control hypertension. Some diuretics may increase the total cholesterol.

Fat One of three types of nutrients that supply energy to the body. Fats contain 9 calories per gram. Fats are found in three different types: saturated, polyunsaturated, and monounsaturated.

Heart Attack Irreversible damage to the heart muscle that results from a decreased or lack of blood supply to a portion of the heart muscle. This is usually caused by atherosclerosis.

Heart Disease Any disease of the heart, including diseases of the muscle, coronary arteries, and valves. The most common type of heart disease is that caused by atherosclerosis, leading to angina or heart attack.

High Density Lipoprotein (HDL) This is the portion of the blood lipids that removes cholesterol and the low density lipoproteins (LDL) from the blood. HDL carries cholesterol and LDL to the liver where it is broken down and excreted from the body. HDL is the "good" fraction of cholesterol. It is desirable to have a high HDL cholesterol value in the blood.

Hydrogenation A process that converts liquid vegetable oil into a more solid product. This process increases the saturated fat content of the product. The more an oil is hydrogenated, the more saturated fat it contains.

Hypercholesterolemia An increase in the cholesterol level in the blood.

Hypertension High blood pressure.

Lipid Any fatty substance that is found in the body. The classification lipid includes cholesterol and triglycerides. Lipids are present in the blood and tissues.

Lipoprotein Lipids that are combined with protein for transport through the blood. Lipoproteins are categorized by their density; LDL are low density and HDL are high density.

Low Density Lipoprotein (LDL) The largest amount of cholesterol is found in the LDL. LDL is deposited in the walls of arteries and is associated with atherosclerosis. LDL is referred to as "bad" cholesterol.

Monounsaturated Fat One type of fat that is available in foods. Monounsaturated fats do not appreciably raise or lower blood cholesterol levels. Olive, canola (rapeseed), and peanut oils are sources of monounsaturated fat.

Polyunsaturated Fat A type of fat that is found in foods of plant origin. Polyunsaturated fats are beneficial in lowering cholesterol levels in the blood. Polyunsaturated fats should be substituted for saturated fats in the diet to help reduce the risk of heart disease. Polyunsaturated fats are mainly found in vegetables and are liquid at room temperature.

Risk Factor A condition that is associated with an increased risk of developing heart disease. These conditions may be genetic traits, habits, or conditions. Some risk factors are: elevated blood cholesterol, hypertension, smoking, male sex, family history, diabetes, obesity, sedentary lifestyle, and increased stress.

Saturated Fat   A fat that is found primarily in foods of animal origin. Saturated fats are also found in products made from palm and coconuts. Saturated fats elevate the blood cholesterol more than any other dietary influence. To help reduce the risk of heart disease, saturated fats should be limited in the diet.

Triglycerides   A type of lipid found in the blood and tissues of the body. Most of the body's fat stores are triglycerides. Elevated blood triglycerides are associated with an increased incidence of heart disease.

Unsaturated Fat   Monounsaturated and polyunsaturated fats are both types of unsaturated fat. Both mono- and poly-unsaturated fats help reduce the cholesterol in the blood and, therefore, reduce the incidence of heart disease. Unsaturated fats are liquid at room temperature.

Index

Vegetable shortening, 11, 16
  substitutes for, 112
Very low density lipoprotein
  (VLDL) cholesterol, nicotinic
  acid and, 75

W
Walnut oil, 43
Water pills. *See* Diuretics
Weight control, 62–67
  alcoholic beverages and, 96
  appetizers and, 92
Weight and height table, 153–154
Whipped cream, low-fat recipe
  for, 121–122

Wine, 96
Women
  cholesterol level recommended
    for, 48, 49, 59
  dietary recommendations for,
    18–20
  lowering cholesterol in, effect
    of, 2n
Worksheets, for daily
  cholesterol/fat intake, 21–23

Y
Yogurt, 26, 45, 137
  frozen, 145